Irritable Bowel Syndrome

Dr Sarah Brewer MA, MB, BChir

IRRITABLE BOWEL SYNDROME

Thorsons
An Imprint of HarperCollins*Publishers*

Thorsons
An Imprint of HarperCollins*Publishers*
77–85 Fulham Palace Road,
Hammersmith, London W6 8JB
1160 Battery Street,
San Francisco, California 94111–1213

Published by Thorsons 1997
10 9 8 7 6 5 4 3 2 1

© Dr Sarah Brewer 1997

Dr Sarah Brewer asserts the moral right to
be identified as the author of this work

A catalogue record for this book
is available from the British Library

ISBN 0 7225 3392 6

Printed and bound in Great Britain by
Caledonian International Book Manufacturing Ltd, Glasgow

To Richard and Saxon

CONTENTS

PREFACE: THE ESSENTIAL GUIDE SERIES

This series offers up-to-date, in-depth information on common health problems. These books contain detailed, medically accurate information in a user-friendly, easy to read style.
Each book covers:

- What the condition is
- How common it is
- Who is affected by it
- Normal body functions and how each condition affects them
- Symptoms
- Causes
- Risk factors
- How the condition is diagnosed – blood tests, investigations, etc.
- Other similar conditions that need to be ruled out
- The drugs used to treat it – including side-effects and who shouldn't take them
- Surgical treatments that can help
- Complementary treatments
- Self-help tips
- Dietary changes that may prove helpful
- Latest research findings
- Addresses of support groups and sources of further information

This invaluable series will answer all your questions and help you to make the best decisions regarding your own health care.

Chapter One

AN INTRODUCTION TO IRRITABLE BOWEL SYNDROME

Irritable bowel syndrome is the most common condition to affect the gut. It is a problem of bowel function rather than structure and, as a result, there is nothing abnormal to find during investigations and no obvious clues to help with the diagnosis. IBS is therefore referred to as a functional disorder rather than an organic one (*see list of definitions at the end of this chapter*). This means that, in the past, the diagnosis of IBS was sometimes an haphazard affair – almost pulled out of a hat, rather than a positive answer as to what was wrong with you.

Despite the lack of physical findings, symptoms experienced by people with IBS can be as severe and disabling as those of any visible organic disease of the gut, and should always be taken seriously – both by yourself and your doctor. Although IBS is not a serious disease in the sense that it does not threaten your life, and is not catching or hereditary, it is serious in that it causes much discomfort and distress.

Lots of research has gone into finding out the cause of IBS, yet the answers are still elusive. There are no specific tests that can pinpoint IBS, but since 1993 new criteria have been drawn up against which your symptoms can be compared. These so-called 'Rome Criteria' (*see below*) have helped doctors to be more scientific about diagnosing the condition and to come up with a more positive, definitive answer. For sufferers, to be told 'Yes, you have irritable bowel syndrome' rather than 'Well, we can't find anything else wrong, therefore you might have IBS' is a big step forward.

The Rome Criteria mean that IBS is no longer a diagnosis of exclusion – one made after more serious bowel disorders have been ruled out. By asking the right questions, and by a careful, physical examination, IBS can now be diagnosed quite confidently on your medical history and by examination alone. This means that fewer patients are subjected to unpleasant tests – with their inevitable worry – to obtain a battery of negative results before being told they have IBS. Referral to hospital for further investigations is now often reserved for more difficult cases: where the diagnosis is unclear, where symptoms suggest an organic problem or where standard treatments have failed.

This advance is a welcome one for the millions of adults who suffer from irritable bowel syndrome throughout the world.

The Rome Criteria

In 1993, an international working team of gastroenterologists defined irritable bowel syndrome as being distinct from other functional disorders of the bowel. In order to diagnose irritable bowel syndrome, there must be *at least three months' continuous or recurrent symptoms of abdominal pain or discomfort which is:*

■ relieved by defecation
■ and/or associated with a change in frequency of passing stool
■ and/or associated with a change in consistency of stool

plus two or more of the following, on at least a quarter of occasions or days:

■ altered stool frequency
■ altered stool form (lumpy/hard or loose/watery)
■ altered stool passage (straining, urgency, or feeling of incomplete evacuation)
■ passage of mucus
■ bloating or feeling of abdominal distension.

Altered stool frequency is usually taken to mean more than three bowel movements per day, or less than three bowel movements per week. Different people, however, have their own individual sense of what is normal for them, and against which changes in bowel habits are measured.

Before the Rome Criteria were drawn up in 1993, doctors relied on an older system of diagnosis known as the Manning Criteria. This had variable success as it was less specific and overlapped with symptoms present in other conditions. According to these less specific Manning Criteria for diagnosing IBS, patients should have three or more of the following symptoms: pain relieved after defecation; more frequent stools after onset of pain; looser stools after onset of pain; abdominal distension; passage of mucus; feeling of incomplete bowel evacuation.

WHAT IS IBS?

The simplest definition is intermittent abdominal discomfort with an alteration in bowel habit for which no cause is found on routine clinical investigation. It is a problem of gut function and seems to be linked with abnormal or exaggerated bowel movements and muscular spasm.

Irritable bowel syndrome is sometimes also known as chronic irritable colon, spastic colon, spastic colitis, spastic constipation, or mucous colitis.

The intestines contract in ordered waves to push food through whilst nutrients and water are absorbed. In IBS, instead of the normal, smooth downward propulsion of bowel contents, their passage is irregular, leading to recurrent symptoms of bloating, wind, constipation, diarrhoea and/or pain.

Imagine the gut as a long, flexible polythene tube filled with porridge which is closed off at one end. If you picked up the closed end of the tube and squeezed it with both hands, the porridge contents would be forced further down the tube. If you moved your hands down the tube, systematically squeezing the porridge further and further down the tube, you would eventually push all the porridge out of the open end of the tube, leaving the tube itself relatively clean and empty.

Now imagine a similar tube filled with porridge, again held with both hands near the closed end. Instead of smoothly constricting the tube in an ordered wave down its length, if you were to let go of the tube with one hand and then randomly squeeze it anywhere you liked along its length, some of the porridge would come out of the tube, but much of it would remain inside, leaving the tube relatively full so it resembled a string of sausages.

In a normally functioning bowel, smooth muscular waves of constriction run down the gut in an ordered fashion. A wave of constriction is preceded by a wave of relaxation, and this pushes the bowel contents downwards. This characteristic movement of the bowel is known as *peristalsis*.

In irritable bowel syndrome, it is thought that peristalsis becomes disordered. Waves of constriction and relaxation become separated and random parts of the bowel may go into cramp. If waves of constriction are speeded up, intestinal 'hurry' – diarrhoea – occurs.

If waves of constriction are slowed down, or become irregular, constipation occurs. This is made worse if the bowel goes into cramp. Constricted bowel contents harden up and more water than normal is re-absorbed by the body. Not surprisingly, this can lead to hardened, concrete-like motions with or without mucus.

If the bowel dilates in between cramp attacks, two things can happen: If the gut is full, the contents become unusually large and difficult to push out; if the gut is empty, it can fill with wind to cause bloating, stretch pains and embarrassing rumblings and escaping wind.

If the bowel stays constricted, and only dilates occasionally, the contents may become concentrated into thin ribbons, or separated into pellets.

One potential problem in diagnosing IBS has been that its symptoms are often similar to those of other gut problems, including inflammatory bowel disease and bowel cancer. As a general rule, if your bowel symptoms develop for the first time over the age of 45, you should be fully investigated to rule out other more potentially serious bowel problems. If your problem is caused by a tumour, for example, you have a good chance of being cured if your symptoms are brought to the attention of a doctor at an early, treatable stage. For this reason, irritable bowel syndrome is not a condition that anyone should try to diagnose themselves.

HOW COMMON IS IBS?

Irritable bowel syndrome is increasingly common. At least a third of the population are affected at some time during their life, even if only mildly. Overall, 15 per cent of people are affected badly enough to consult their doctor. This figure is surprisingly constant throughout the world. Studies in the UK, US, France, New Zealand and China suggest that irritable bowel syndrome is present in 11–20 per cent of adults at any one time, although not all consult a doctor about their symptoms. It is thought to be less common among inhabitants of parts of Africa and Asia – possibly because of the high amount of roughage in their diet.

IBS is the commonest gut problem seen in hospital gastroenterology clinics, where it accounts for between 40 and 50 per cent of out-patient referrals. Many more patients are known to suffer in silence, either putting up with their symptoms because they believe little can be done to help, or because they are too embarrassed to talk about bowel problems. Significant numbers of people are also thought to have learned how to control their symptoms through dietary and lifestyle changes, without ever seeking help from their doctor. This is not ideal, however. Because so many potentially serious bowel problems can produce a similar picture, it is important that a diagnosis of IBS should be made by a doctor after a full consideration of your symptoms and a full physical examination, including a digital rectal examination (*see page 105*).

WHO GETS IT?

IBS is traditionally said to affect young and middle-aged adults – especially women. Symptoms usually start between the ages of 15 and 40, with the commonest presentation being between the ages of 30 and 40. It can affect anyone at any age, however, and new data suggests that more people are affected in the 45–65 age range than in younger age-groups.

Researchers have recently found that people with IBS are more likely to have suffered from abdominal pain in childhood.

These recurrent attacks are often dismissed as 'growing pains' and are eventually forgotten by parents, but it is possible that as many as 1 in 6 older children has symptoms of IBS (*see page 55*).

Is IBS More Common in Women?

Traditionally, IBS was seen as a problem affecting women rather than men. Studies now suggest that men are just as likely to have symptoms of IBS as women, but are less likely to consult their doctor and be labelled as having IBS. As a result, two out of every three sufferers who are referred to a hospital clinic and diagnosed as having IBS are female. This leads many researchers automatically to label IBS as psychosomatic and to link it with hysteria and neurosis. More enlightened scientists, however, started wondering about the role of the female hormones oestrogen and progesterone in IBS (*see page 51*).

IS THERE A CURE?

Despite active research, the exact cause of IBS remains unknown and therefore a cure is still elusive. However, dietary and lifestyle changes can help to relieve symptoms in many cases (more details about this are in Chapter 10), and drugs are often helpful in controlling bothersome symptoms such as recurrent diarrhoea or constipation (as discussed in Chapter 8).

Many sufferers find that their symptoms improve with time and disappear in later life. One study found that after five years, 70 per cent of sufferers were free of symptoms. This fits in with the observation that it is rare to see an elderly patient who has IBS.

One surgeon may have stumbled across a permanent cure for IBS. He found that patients undergoing a new, modified surgical treatment for piles (haemorrhoids) lost their IBS symptoms. This might be due to the cutting of small nerves which prevented feedback hyperstimulation of the gut triggered by spasm in the rectum. If these findings are validated by formal trials, this operation may provide a cure for people with disabling symptoms (*see page 126*).

DEFINITIONS

Functional Disorder
A problem caused by abnormal function – with no obvious anatomical or physiological abnormality to explain it. A functional disorder is often interpreted as a psychosomatic disease and sufferers may be inappropriately labelled as neurotic. IBS diagnoses are now moving away from these negative connotations.

Organic Disorder
A problem with an obvious anatomical or physiological abnormality to explain it, such as bowel stricture, bowel cancer or diverticular disease.

Psychosomatic Disease
An illness resulting from the effects of excessive or repressed emotions upon bodily function. For example, a tension headache brought on by stress.

Functional Gastrointestinal Disorder
A variable combination of unexplained, chronic or recurrent gastrointestinal symptoms not explained by structural or biochemical abnormalities. These may include symptoms attributable to the mouth and throat (oropharynx), gullet (oesophagus), stomach, bile duct system (biliary tree), small or large intestine, or the anus. Examples include non-ulcer dyspepsia (indigestion) and irritable bowel syndrome.

Functional Bowel Disorder
A functional gastrointestinal disorder with symptoms attributable to the mid or lower intestinal tract. The symptoms include abdominal pain, bloating or distension with various symptoms of disordered defecation.

Syndrome
A group of symptoms and/or signs which together form a recognizable pattern or symptom complex typical of a particular disease.

Disease
An abnormality of structure or function in any part of the body (other than those arising from injury). It is diagnosed by a characteristic set of signs or symptoms and in most cases, its cause, pathology and future outcomes are known.

Chapter Two

THE NORMAL BOWEL

To understand how some of the symptoms of IBS develop, it is worth looking at the function and muscular activity of the normal bowel.

The gastrointestinal tract is a long tube which starts at the mouth and ends at the anal sphincter. It is basically a food processing system that accepts complex food molecules at one end and breaks these down into simpler, soluble nutritional components which are absorbed into the bloodstream. Waste products are disposed of – usually in neat packages – at the other end.

A combination of mechanical and chemical disruption breaks food down as it passes through the intestinal tract:

■ mechanical – muscles in the stomach wall produce a churning motion that mixes food, while co-ordinated contractions throughout the tract (peristalsis) push the gut contents downwards
■ chemical – acids, alkalis and enzymes secreted by glands in the wall of the gut and associated organs (such as the liver and pancreas) dissolve chemical bonds and break complex food molecules down into simpler ones.

Digestion starts in the mouth, where biting and chewing reduces food into suitable portions for swallowing. The food is also moistened in the mouth by saliva. Saliva contains enzymes (molecules that trigger chemical reactions or speed them up) which start to digest starch. The tongue then rolls the food into a ball (bolus) ready for swallowing.

The swallowing reflex is triggered when food reaches the back of your throat. This reflex is co-ordinated by centres in the

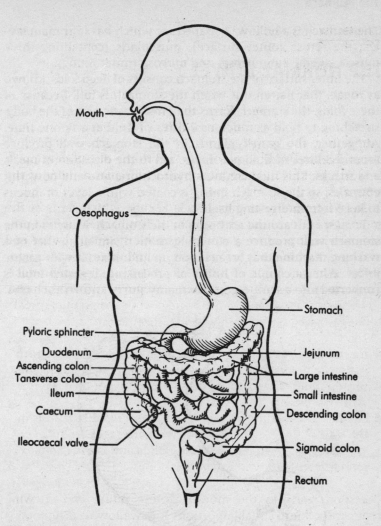

Mouth

Oesophagus

Stomach

Pyloric sphincter

Duodenum

Ascending colon

Tansverse colon

Ileum

Caecum

Ileocaecal valve

Jejunum

Large intestine

Small intestine

Descending colon

Sigmoid colon

Rectum

The gastrointestinal tract

brain stem which initiate an automatic wave of muscle contraction to propel food down the oesophagus (gullet), which links the mouth and stomach.

The Stomach

The stomach is a hollow, J-shaped sac which has four main layers: the serosa (outer surface), muscularis (containing three muscle layers), submucosa, and mucosa (inner lining).

The inner surface of the stomach consists of deep folds, known as rugae, that flatten out when the stomach is full. Because of these folds, the stomach forms the most elastic part of the body, stretching to hold as much as 2 litres of fluid at any one time. Altogether, the gastric glands in the stomach wall produce around 3 litres of fluid per day to aid in the digestion of meals and snacks. This fluid contains hydrochloric acid and powerful enzymes, so the stomach lining is coated with a layer of mucus to keep it from digesting itself.

Food spends around six hours in the stomach. Muscles in the stomach wall produce a churning motion similar to that of a washing machine that breaks food up and mixes it with gastric juices. After a couple of hours of processing, ingested food is converted into a semi-digested, creamy slurry known as chyme.

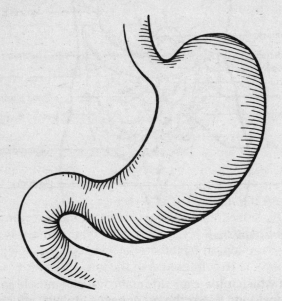

The stomach

The exit to the stomach is guarded by a powerful ring of muscle called the pyloric sphincter. This is usually kept tightly closed to keep the stomach contents in. Once digestion is well on its way, regular, wave-like contractions in the muscular wall of the stomach start to push stomach contents downwards towards the pyloric sphincter. The ring of muscle then relaxes for a few seconds to let a small quantity of chyme squirt through into the next part of the gut, the duodenum.

The duodenum forms the first part of the small intestines. As more and more semi-digested food passes into the duodenum, the stomach gradually shrinks down in size as it empties.

The Small Intestines

The small intestines, or foregut, are highly coiled to fit into the abdominal cavity. They form a tube around 285 cm long and 3.5 cm in diameter. This part of the bowel is usually in a semi-contracted state with a high muscular tone. This is well illustrated by the fact that, after death, when the muscles lining the small intestine relax, the tube more than doubles in length to 7 m long. Abnormal contraction or distension of the small bowel can cause symptoms of *primary foregut motility disorder* – one of the three newly identified variants of IBS (*see page 22*).

As mentioned, the first part of the small intestine after the stomach is the duodenum. This is a curved, ⊏-shaped tube around 25 cm long that is fixed to the back wall of the abdominal cavity. It leads into the next part of the gut, the ileum. The intestinal juices secreted into the duodenum are alkaline, to neutralize acidity from the stomach. Bile from the liver and powerful enzymes from the pancreas also flow into the duodenum to start the next phase of digestion.

Like the stomach, the walls of the small (and large) intestines have three muscle layers: an outer, longitudinal layer that runs down the length of the gut; a middle, circular layer that runs around the circumference of the gut; and an inner, longitudinal layer.

These layers are sandwiched between the inner mucous lining of the bowel (mucosa) and the outer coating (serosa).

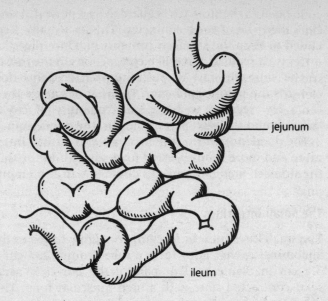

jejunum

ileum

The small intestines

When longitudinal muscle contracts, the bowel length shortens. When circular muscle contracts, the bore of the gut narrows. It is the ordered, co-ordinated contraction of these muscle layers that pushes food down through the tract.

The jejunum is the name given to the first 40 per cent of small intestine below the duodenum, while the ileum is the next 60 per cent. There is no distinct border between the two and this division is somewhat arbitrary.

As food travels down it is mixed with intestinal juices (succus entericus) secreted by mucosal glands.

The inner lining of the small intestines is covered in tiny projections around 1 mm long, called villi. These increase the surface area of the intestinal wall to speed up absorption of the products of digestion, including vitamins and fluid. Nutrients pass into the villi where they enter tiny blood capillaries for transportation to the liver, or into small lymph vessels, called lacteals, for distribution into the lymph system. The small intestines process around 9 litres of fluid per day – 2 litres from your diet and 7 litres secreted in the form of digestive juices. Only 1–2 litres of fluid are passed through into the large bowel, however; the rest is absorbed in the small intestines.

By the time food has reached the end of the small intestines and passes into the large bowel, the process of digestion is complete. The junction between the small and large bowel – the ileocaecal valve – is formed by the narrower ileum protruding into the much wider large intestine. This arrangement means that an increase in pressure in the large bowel squeezes the valve closed, while increases in pressure in the small intestine lets it open. This allows intestinal contents to pass from the small to the large bowel, but not in the reverse direction. The ileocaecal valve is normally closed, but every time a peristaltic wave of contraction reaches it, it opens briefly to let some chyme squirt through into the upper portion of the large intestines (the caecum).

The Large Intestines

The large intestines, also known as the hind gut or large bowel, form a wide tube that is around 1 m long. Like the small intestines, it usually has a high muscular tone and relaxes to measure 1.5 m long after death. The first part of the large bowel, the colon, is shaped rather like a loose, floppy M with a flattened cross-piece. It is made up of five main parts: the caecum, ascending colon, transverse colon, descending colon, and sigmoid colon.

The colon starts with a pouch, the caecum, into which the ileocaecal valve protrudes. At the base of the caecum, the appendix – which has no known function in humans – branches off as a narrow, blind alley. The caecum leads into the ascending colon, which travels up the right-hand side of the abdomen. The transverse colon passes across the top of the abdominal cavity and leads into the descending colon down the left-hand side. The final part forms a curve, the sigmoid colon, which connects with the rectum.

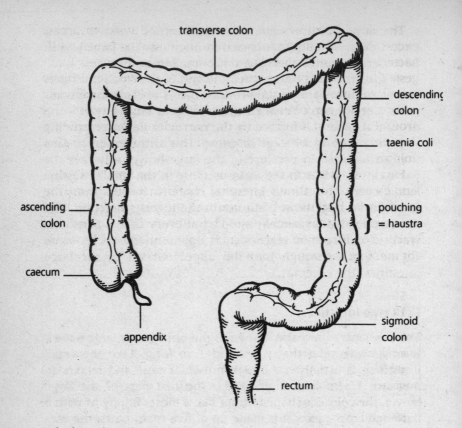

transverse colon

descending colon

taenia coli

pouching = haustra

ascending colon

caecum

appendix

sigmoid colon

rectum

The large intestines

The three muscle layers of the gut are arranged differently in the large bowel compared with those in the stomach and small intestines. The outer, longitudinal layer of muscle fibres are collected together into three longitudinal bands known as the taenia coli. Because these bands are shorter than the rest of the colon, they act rather like drawstrings to draw the colonic wall into out-pouchings known as haustra. The lining of the large bowel (mucosa) is also different from that found in the small intestines – it does not contain villi, and only contains colonic glands that secrete lubricating mucus. Mucus production is mainly stimulated by the mechanical contact of faeces with the colon wall.

The large intestines are mainly concerned with absorbing excess fluid, salts and minerals from the bowel contents, while bacterial fermentation helps to break down and process undigested fibre. After passing through the large bowel, semi-liquid bowel contents are usually transformed into solidified waste matter as 90 per cent of their fluid content is absorbed – of around 2 litres of bowel contents received into the colon each day, only around 200–250 ml of semi-solid waste remains for voiding.

Finally, food enters the last part of the large bowel, the rectum for expulsion through the anal canal. Normally the rectum is empty as distension of this part of the gut triggers a large voiding reflex that takes you to the bathroom. Abnormal contraction or distension of the rectum is thought to be responsible for many of the symptoms of IBS.

SOME OF THE IMPORTANT ENZYMES FOUND IN THE DIGESTIVE TRACT

Region/Gland	Secretion	Enzymes	Food Acted On	Product
mouth/salivary glands	saliva	amylase	starch	maltose
stomach	gastric juices	pepsins, lipase	proteins, fats	amino and fatty acids
pancreas	pancreatic juices	trypsin, elastase, lipase, amylase	proteins, fats, starch	amino acids, fatty acids, maltose
small intestine	succus entericus	sucrase, lactase, peptidases, lipase	sucrose, lactose, proteins, fats	fructose, glucose, galactose, amino and fatty acids
colon	bacterial secretions	bacterial enzymes	undigested vegetable fibre	gases and fermentation products

Intestinal Contractions

Peristalsis

Contraction of the small intestine is co-ordinated by waves of electrical activity. These start in the circular layer of smooth muscle in the duodenum and pass downwards. This is known as the *small bowel slow wave*, and as it goes through the jejunum it has a frequency of around 12 contractions per minute (about as often as you breath in and out at rest). The wave then slows slightly, so that contractions in the ileum occur around nine times per minute. This slowing is partly because the volume of intestinal contents decreases as intestinal contents pass down and fluid and nutrients are absorbed.

Peristalsis involves the co-ordinated contraction and relaxation of the circular muscle layer running round the bowel. Two waves of muscle activity are involved: a wave of dilation closely followed by a wave of contraction. As the wave of contraction runs down the bowel, it pushes food ahead of it along the digestive tract into the dilated area. In other words, one section of bowel constricts while the neighbouring region beyond it dilates, so that food is pushed from the constricted area into the dilated area. The dilated area then contracts and the next region along relaxes, so that food is pushed further down the tract.

Peristalsis within the colon is co-ordinated by a wave of electrical activity called the *slow wave of the colon*. Unlike the similar wave passing through the small intestine, the peristaltic activity in the colon gets faster as it passes along the colon. At the caecum, the wave occurs at a rate of around two contractions per minute, while at the sigmoid colon it reaches a speed of six contractions per minute.

Segmental Contractions

Another type of contraction also occurs in the normal gut. This is known as segmentation contraction and, as its name implies, involves ring-like contractions of parts of the gut. These come and go at fairly regular intervals, to be replaced by another set of ring contractions in the segments between the previous constrictions. These actions move intestinal contents (chyme) to and fro so that as many nutrients as possible come into contact with the bowel wall for absorption.

Mass Action Contraction
A third type of contraction occurs only in the colon – the so-called mass action contraction. This triggers simultaneous constriction of smooth muscle over large areas of the colon, which moves large bowel motions from one part of the colon to another. These waves of activity also move dryish material into the rectum. Rectal filling and distension then trigger the desire to open your bowels (defecation reflex).

Myenteric Reflex

If the intestinal wall becomes stretched at any point (such as through wind distension) it triggers a new reflex wave of deep circular muscle contraction. This forms behind the point of stimulation and passes down the intestine towards the rectum at a rate that varies from 2 to as much as 25 cm per second. This stretch response is called the myenteric (intestinal muscle) reflex. This differs from a normal peristaltic wave in that it is not preceded by the normal wave of relaxation. The waves also vary in their intensity and in the distance they travel. Very intense waves, known as peristaltic rushes, happen when the bowel is obstructed.

Gastrocolic and Gastroileal Reflexes

As food distends the stomach, a hormone called cholecystokinin (CCK) is secreted in the duodenum. This causes the colon and rectum to contract and often brings on a strong desire to open the bowels (gastrocolic reflex). When food leaves the stomach and the stomach shrinks, the caecum relaxes slightly (gastroileal reflex). This lets some chyme through and further stimulates activity within the large bowel. Both these reflexes are thought to play a part in those with IBS who develop discomfort, pain or a need to visit the toilet after eating.

Defecation Reflex

When the rectum becomes distended with faeces, reflex contractions of its muscular walls stimulate a powerful urge to open the bowels. The internal part of the anal sphincter relaxes while the outer part – which is usually under voluntary control – stays tightly shut until you allow it to open. Evolution has kindly arranged things so that normally, as moderate pressure within the rectum increases, the tighter the external anal sphincter becomes to prevent unwanted accidents.

The urge to defecate is usually first felt when pressure within the rectum reaches 18 mm Hg. When pressure increases to around 55 mm Hg, the inevitable occurs and the external sphincter opens, whether you wish it or not, to expel the contents of the rectum. At pressures beneath this extreme, voluntary voiding can occur by relaxing the external anal sphincter and tensing the abdominal muscles (straining).

NORMAL BOWEL MOTIONS

Strangely, bowel emptying is one of the least understood and least studied of all normal body functions despite the amount of grief it can cause. While some people normally open their bowels once every two or three days, others defecate once daily, and some regularly pass motions as often as three times a day. According to one study involving almost 2,000 people, the commonest bowel habit was once daily. In general, however, bowel habits were found to be quite irregular. Women seemed to suffer more from constipated-type stools and irregular bowel habit than men. Women were more likely to open their bowels less than three times per week, while defecating more than twice a day was more common in males. Most people in the study defecated in the morning, soon after waking up.

The study concluded that there are differences in bowel habit between men and women, and between women of childbearing age and those who are post-menopausal. A general finding was that bowel transit time is slower in women, especially younger ones. Surprisingly, it seemed that the commonly accepted normal bowel habit of voiding once a day was actually less common than expected.

It seems that frequency of defecation is a poor guide to how well your gut is functioning. It is much more useful to assess stool form and consistency, as these bear a closer relationship to how long food stays in your intestines (bowel transit time), and to measure daily faecal weight.

It is an alteration in bowel movements that is important in diagnosing irritable bowel syndrome and other gastrointestinal disorders. Altered stool frequency is usually taken to mean more than three bowel movements per day, or less than three bowel movements per week in someone who normally has a different pattern of bowel frequency. Different people, of course, have their own individual sense of what is normal for them. Interestingly, however, when bowel activity is independently monitored it seems that many people exaggerate their bowel frequency by three or more stools per week.

Stool Form and Consistency

A team of gastroenterologists in Bristol have drawn up a stool classification scale which defines seven different types of bowel motion:

Type 1: Separate hard lumps, like nuts
Type 2: Sausage-shaped but lumpy
Type 3: Like a sausage or snake but with cracks on the surface
Type 4: Like a sausage or snake, smooth and soft
Type 5: Soft blobs with clear-cut edges
Type 6: Fluffy pieces with ragged edges, a mushy stool
Type 7: Watery, no solid pieces.

Types 3 and 4 are described as perfectly normal bowel motions.
Types 1, 6 and 7 are considered abnormal and suggest a current bowel problem or increased risk of developing one in future.
Types 1 and 2 are abnormally hard (that is, constipation) and result from a slow bowel transit time. These seem to be linked with an increased risk of gallstones.

Type 5 is poorly formed, soft and verging on abnormal.
Types 6 and 7 are abnormally loose (that is, diarrhoea).

It is not always that easy to assess your stool form, however. It is a peculiarity of British toilet bowls that they are designed so the stools virtually sink out of sight, compared to toilet bowls in the rest of Europe or the US, which allow stool-gazing to become a finer art.

Straining

Straining – contraction of the diaphragm and abdominal muscles, with a tensed, closed throat – used to be thought of as a natural and necessary habit in everyone. It is now known to be associated with the type of stool passed – the lumpier the stool (that is, stool Types 1 and 2) the more likely it is that you will need to strain to pass it out. Frequent straining is therefore a good indication that constipation is present. Studies suggest that straining is more common in women than men, and that on average women strain to start one out of every three (32 per cent) defecations, and strain to finish 15 per cent of defecations. Men strain to start one out of every four to five defecations (22 per cent), and strain to finish 9 per cent of defecations.

Many people seem to strain even when passing soft or mushy unformed stools (Types 5 and 6), so it seems likely that straining in some people is just a habit. Recurrent straining may trigger a number of other problems, including haemorrhoids (piles), hiatus hernia, inguinal hernia, diverticular disease of the colon (out-pouchings of the bowel wall), and possibly even varicose veins.

Bowel Bacteria

Normally, the contents of the first part of the small bowel, the jejunum, are virtually sterile. This is probably due to the digestive enzymes present, and the fact that chyme passes through relatively quickly. A few bacteria are found in the ileum (as well as Candida yeast cells in 50 per cent of people), but it is not until the colon that lots of bacteria are seen. These bowel bacteria are usually beneficial, in that they:

- ferment and help to break down undigested fibre
- bulk up the stools to make defecation easier – over half the weight of your stools consists of bacteria
- compete for nutrients with potentially harmful bacteria and yeasts to stop them overgrowing
- make acids and natural antibiotics/antifungal substances which inhibit growth of other organisms
- make and secrete vitamin K, B-group vitamins, biotin and folic acid, which can be absorbed and used in the body
- absorb some cholesterol and fatty acids from the gut, preventing their reabsorption – when some antibiotics are given, blood cholesterol levels (especially of the more harmful LDL-cholesterol) can go up.

Stools are usually slightly acid (pH 5–7) due to the presence of acids made by bacteria.

Substances formed by bacterial metabolism – mainly indole and skatole – are largely responsible for the characteristic odour of faeces. The brown colour of the stools is due to pigments formed when bowel bacteria interact with bile. If bile is prevented from entering the gut (if for example as a result of a blocked bile duct), the stools will be pale or even white.

Bacteria frequently found in the stools include:

- Escherichia coli
- Enterobacter aerogenes
- Bacteroides fragilis
- Streptococcus faecalis
- Clostridium sp.

Stools contain:

- water: 75 per cent
- solids: 25 per cent
  - Of which:
  - around 30 per cent = bacteria and yeasts
  - around 15 per cent = inorganic material (such as calcium and phosphates)
  - around 5 per cent = fats
  - a varying amount is undigested plant fibre (roughage) depending on diet
- a small amount of desquamated (shed) bowel lining cells, mucus and digestive enzymes

Chapter Three

THE IRRITABLE BOWEL

It is not that long ago that doctors regarded IBS as a preoccupation with, and excessive concern about, normal intestinal events. Eminent gastroenterologists blithely claimed that it was unclear to what extent 'irritable bowel syndrome is a normal perception of abnormal events, or an abnormal perception of normal events'.

It was not until a study carried out as recently as 1991 that this point was settled. Researchers studied bowel habit and defecation for a month in 26 patients with diagnosed IBS, 27 women with recurrent colonic pain who had not consulted a doctor, and 27 women with apparently normal bowels. Surprisingly, abdominal pain and bloating occurred in most of the so-called normal women. However, compared with normal subjects, the researchers found that the women with IBS:

- suffered pain six times more frequently, and that this pain was more often described as severe
- bloating occurred three times more often
- defecation was more likely to be frequent, irregular and to have an erratic form
- urgency was four times more frequent
- straining to defecate was nine times more common and often associated with feelings of incomplete evacuation.

The authors concluded that 'Patients with the irritable bowel syndrome have real cause for complaint and their bowel function is truly abnormal.' They also stated that 'Patients with the irritable bowel syndrome are sometimes accused of being obsessed with their bowels. But who can blame them when their defecations start suddenly and unpredictably and finish slowly and uncertainly?"[1]

In IBS, bowel function differs from normal in the ways defined by the Rome Criteria (*see page 2*). The basic abnormality in IBS seems to be a disturbance of muscle contraction in the gut, but no physiological, muscular or nerve ending abnormality has yet been found to account for this.

ABNORMAL GUT MOTILITY IN IBS

The term irritable bowel syndrome is misleading, in that the bowel is not so much irritable as prone to bouts of sluggish/ lethargic behaviour, overactivity, or both.

Bowel motility studies in the 1960s suggested that in some people with constipation, the colon was more active, with stronger, more frequent contractions which were less effective in moving bowel contents on. As a result, stool passage was held up and abdominal pain occurred as a result of colonic cramping. In contrast, patients with diarrhoea seemed to have less contractions, which were weaker, and therefore did not hold up the passage of stool. The lower portion of the colon (sigmoid) seemed to act more like a valve than a processing unit for absorbing excess fluid. These researchers developed a colon motility index (frequency of colon contractions multiplied by their strength) to reflect this, but unfortunately this index did not prove to be a very accurate way of predicting constipation or diarrhoea.

In the 1970s, it was noted that patients with IBS were more likely than non-sufferers to have regular muscle electrical activity at a frequency of three cycles/minute throughout the bowel. Constipation seemed to be linked with short bursts of this electrical activity in the colon, while diarrhoea was associated with lack of electrical activity.

The 1980s brought the realization that dysfunction (both of secretion and contraction patterns) in the small intestines was also probably involved in some patients with IBS, especially in some of the responses – especially diarrhoea – to stress hormones. A series of experiments in which balloons were inflated in different places within the gut also identified particular trigger points that could bring on abdominal pain characteristic of IBS in most sufferers.

The 1990s brought the finding that patients with IBS experience bowel pain when their intestines – especially the rectum – were inflated with gas to a much lower pressure than that tolerated by other people, although their pain thresholds elsewhere in the body seemed to be the same. Pain sensitivity in the gut seems to be greater in IBS sufferers than non-sufferers. Recently it was also found that bowel contents move through the small intestines faster in patients with IBS than those without.

Most researchers now believe that IBS is due to an abnormality of bowel contraction or motility. What actually causes this is unknown, although it seems to be linked to malfunctioning of part of the nervous system supplying the gut.

Much of the bowel's motility seems to be controlled by a particular nerve chemical (neurotransmitter) called serotonin. This is also sometimes referred to as 5-hydroxytryptamine (5-HT). It is possible that the diarrhoea found in IBS is due to increased amounts of serotonin in nerve endings, while constipation is linked with a fall in serotonin levels. This has yet to be proved, however. Certainly treatment with a drug that increases availability of serotonin at nerve endings has been shown to result in a more rapid movement of bowel contents through the intestines, leading to diarrhoea.

When you eat, a hormone called cholecystokinin (CCK) is released from cells in the lining of the upper small intestine (duodenum). This stimulates contraction of the colon and is thought to trigger the gastrocolic reflex which often makes you want to open your bowels after a meal – this reflex is very obvious in young babies. Another possibility, therefore, is that IBS results from an abnormal response to CCK. One study found that people with IBS experience more pain than non-sufferers when CCK was given by injection; this finding is currently undergoing further investigation.

All these studies have led to the conclusion that IBS is linked with over-sensitivity of both the small and large intestines to different stimuli such as drugs, stress, distension and the normal events of digestion, absorption and the passage of food through the gut. Having said that, it's worth pointing out that some gastroenterologists still feel that a bowel condition affecting at least 11 per cent of an otherwise physically healthy adult population may not be an abnormality at all. The symptoms may form one end of the spectrum of what is essentially normal bowel function.

1 Heaton, K. W., Ghosh, S., Braddon, F. E.M., 'How bad are the symptoms and bowel dysfunction of patients with the irritable bowel syndrome? A prospective, controlled study with emphasis on stool form', *Gut* 32.1 (1991): 73–9.

Chapter Four

SYMPTOMS

The symptoms of IBS vary from person to person and may come and go over a period of time. The ones that occur most often include:

- lower abdominal pain or discomfort
- bloating
- wind – distension, rumblings (borborygmi) and flatulence
- constipation
- diarrhoea
- urgency (having to rush to the loo)
- altered stool frequency
- altered stool form
- altered stool passage with feelings of incomplete emptying
- mucus in the stool
- nausea
- upper abdominal pain
- rectal pain.

Researchers at the Central Middlesex Hospital NHS Trust have identified three different types of IBS based on the main symptoms experienced by sufferers: spastic colon syndrome, functional diarrhoea syndrome, and primary foregut motility disorder.

SPASTIC COLON SYNDROME

Spastic colon syndrome is where the onset of lower abdominal pain is associated with:

■ passing looser stools than normal
■ abdominal distension
■ relief of symptoms on opening the bowels
■ feelings of incomplete evacuation of the bowel
■ mucus in the stools.

Loose motions and constipation tend to alternate. Females suffering from this form of IBS are more likely to report difficulty in passing urine and gynaecological problems, with IBS symptoms being worse at certain times of the menstrual cycle. Spastic colon syndrome is the classic form of IBS, due to abnormal contractility of the large bowel. Constipation is usually a major feature of spastic colon syndrome, and tends to respond well to an increase of fibre in the diet. Smooth muscle relaxant drugs and anti-spasmodics are usually helpful too.

FUNCTIONAL DIARRHOEA SYNDROME

Functional diarrhoea syndrome is associated with:

■ increased frequency of bowel movements
■ urgency (having to rush to the bathroom)
■ passing several stools in rapid succession, often in the morning
■ stools that characteristically become looser and looser throughout the day.

Sufferers are frequently left exhausted and tired, and the rapidity with which the bowels have to be opened can mean that they are housebound or unable to travel far. This form of IBS is likely to be made worse by following a high-fibre diet, but will usually respond to treatment with anti-diarrhoeals such as loperamide or immodium.

PRIMARY FOREGUT MOTILITY DISORDER

Primary foregut motility disorder is linked with:

- abdominal pain which is usually right-sided
- bloating, which may be so severe that you have to wear loose clothing or even wear several different sizes of clothes over several days
- feeling full after eating only a small amount of food
- poor appetite
- sometimes weight loss.

There is usually no significant disturbance of bowel habit in this type of IBS, so that diarrhoea or constipation are not a major problem. This disorder of the foregut is in fact due to abnormal contraction of the small intestine rather than of the colon. It seems to affect women more than men. Unfortunately, the condition can be difficult to treat, although drugs that stimulate and regulate intestinal motility (such as cisapride) may help.

This is not a fool-proof classification of classic IBS types, however. Many people cannot fit their symptoms neatly into one group or another.

MOST FREQUENT SYMPTOMS

Pain

The pain of IBS is usually cramp-like or colicky and comes and goes in waves. It can be felt anywhere in the abdomen but is often worse on the lower, left-hand side – except in the primary foregut motility disorder, when bloating is more often linked with pain on the right. The pain may worsen after eating, as this stimulates contraction of the colon (gastrocolic reflex). Sufferers usually find that opening the bowels or passing wind brings relief.

The abdominal pain experienced in IBS seems to be a combination of stretch (distension pain) and spasm (constriction pain). Research has shown that by introducing a balloon into the bowel and periodically inflating it within the intestinal tract, from top to bottom, the pain and discomfort produced are similar to that experienced in IBS, implying that distension may be the main factor.

When balloons are inflated at different sites in the colon, pain is felt in different parts of the abdomen by different people, so it is difficult to tell which part of the colon is in spasm in each sufferer. Just because pain is felt in the upper abdomen, for example, this doesn't mean that the pain is coming from the underlying transverse part of the colon. Nerves from the gut pass pack to the spinal cord and also supply other parts of the abdominal cavity on the way. This may lead to referred pain, in which pain coming from the bowel is interpreted by the brain as coming from the back, for instance. This is the same principle as when pain from the heart (angina) is felt running down the left arm, or pain from the gallbladder is felt in the tip of the right shoulder.

If spasm occurs high in the gut, it can lead to nausea, whereas if it occurs lower down, it is more likely to cause constipation as it interferes with the propulsion of food through the colon and slows down bowel transit time. This allows more fluid to be absorbed, with constipation the result.

Distension or Bloating

Distension is often the most troublesome symptom of IBS. For some reason, distension seem to be worse in women than in men. It seems to be triggered by eating, and typically gets worse as the day progresses. Many women find they need to loosen their clothing in the late afternoon and often tell embarrassed tales about being mistakenly congratulated for pregnancy.

Bloating seems to be associated with two of the three recently identified variants of IBS: the spastic colon syndrome and primary motility disorder of the foregut.

Several theories have been suggested to account for the abdominal distension, including:

- excess intra-abdominal gas
- flattening out (downward depression) of the diaphragm

- protrusion of the abdominal wall due to poor muscle tone
- exaggerated spinal curve (lumbar lordosis)
- fluid retention.

Initial results of measuring abdominal girth with CAT scan, estimation of abdominal gas and measurement of lumbar spine angles have suggested that the main reason was excess gas. A later study, however, suggested that the cause was not a build-up of gas, but a forward protrusion of the front abdominal wall, although without any change in the diaphragm or spinal curve.

There is no doubt that distension does occur, and that it seems to be due to disordered intestinal motility or contraction. It is worth remembering that the small intestines form a tube around 2.85 metres long and that it has a high muscle tone (that is, the muscle fibres are normally partially contracted). After death, when the muscles lining the small intestine relax, the tube more than doubles in length to 7 m long. It may well be that excessive and abnormal relaxation of the small intestines may occur throughout the day, lengthening the gut so that it occupies more space, leading to abdominal distension.

Wind

Wind (flatus) is a common symptom in IBS, and excessive flatulence often accompanies abdominal pain and bloating. It burbles around causing pain, distension and embarrassing noises (borborygmi) until escaping – upwards through the mouth, or downwards through the anus – suddenly and sometimes explosively. In general, wind in the stomach is expelled upwards by burping, while wind in the small intestines and colon is expelled via the anus. Bowel gases come from several different sources, such as the gas present in fizzy drinks, air swallowed with food, air swallowed nervously by some people (aerophagia), and gases released during bacterial fermentation of fibre in the large bowel.

Because the intestines are not contracting properly in IBS, it used to be thought that air swallowed naturally during eating and drinking was the cause of the problem. This is not the case, however, as analysis of the gas shows that only a small fraction comes from the atmosphere. Most intestinal gas comes from colonic bacteria breaking down indigestible fibre and starches not absorbed in the small intestines. The bacteria do this through a process of fermentation which releases short-chain fatty acids, heat, and gases such as hydrogen, carbon dioxide, methane and sometimes foul-smelling sulphur-containing gases such as hydrogen sulphide. This excess gas cannot be reabsorbed to any great extent, although some passes into the bloodstream and is excreted through the lungs. A small amount is used up in other bacterial metabolic reactions, but around 1–2.5 litres per day is expelled through the rectum.

Surprisingly, there is no evidence that patients with IBS produce more intestinal gases than people without symptoms. Research suggests that most people pass gas 12–20 times per day. Similarly, the make-up of flatus gases is no different in people with IBS than in others – and the amount of residual gas remaining in the bowels at any one time is similar (up to 200 ml). Some differences have been noticed, however. Wind passes through the gut of people with IBS more slowly than in those without symptoms, and sufferers seem to be more sensitive to the distension it causes. The gas is also more likely to pass backwards through the bowel and to reflux up into the stomach to be expelled by burping. Wind symptoms, therefore, seem to be due to abnormal motility of the intestines and disordered passage of wind through the gut, rather than to the production of excess gas.

It is worth mentioning that some people lack the right enzymes to digest certain foods, especially dairy foods which require enzymes such as lactase to break down milk sugar (lactose). Inadequate amounts of lactase lead to lactose intolerance, which can produce wind and loose bowels. These people will find their symptoms improve dramatically on cutting out milk-based products from their diet (*see Chapter 10*).

Some foods contain compounds that increase gas production in everyone, however. Beans, for example, contain substances such as raffinose. Soaking beans overnight before cooking will help to aid their digestion and decrease flatulence.

If you are prone to excessive flatus:

- Try avoiding foods that promote bacterial fermentation and gas production such as beans, lentils, cauliflower, cabbage, broccoli, Brussels sprouts and cucumber.
- Eat meals slowly, chewing each mouthful thoroughly.
- Avoid food or drinks that are too hot.
- Avoid fizzy drinks.
- Avoid chewing gum and sucking boiled sweets.
- Try drinking herbal teas containing camomile, fennel, ginger, sage or peppermint.
- Try charcoal tablets or biscuits, which absorb unpleasant flatus odours and excess gas.
- Try Windcheaters – available in chemists – containing simethicone (activated dimethicone).

FLATUS-FORMING FOODS

- beans
- lentils
- milk and milk products
- onions
- celery
- carrots
- cabbage, broccoli, Brussels sprouts
- raisins
- bananas
- apricots
- wheatgerm

THE CHEMICALS PRESENT IN BOWEL GAS (FLATUS)

- nitrogen
- carbon dioxide
- hydrogen
- methane
- hydrogen sulphide
- methanethiol
- dimethyl sulphide

Not all flatus contains sulphur-containing (smelly) compounds all the time – the reasons are currently under investigation.

If no gas is passed through the rectum over a prolonged period of time (such as 24 hours), you may have a bowel blockage – especially if other symptoms such as pain, distension and absolute constipation (not opening the bowels at all) are present. If this happens, call a doctor straightaway.

Constipation

Most doctors define constipation as passing bowel motions less than twice a week, or straining at stool more than 25 per cent of the time. Constipation is a common and distressing feature of IBS and occurs more often than diarrhoea. It is made worse by uncoordinated contractions and spasm of the muscular bowel walls, which squashes bowel contents rather than pushing them through. As a result, the bowels may not open for days at a time – so-called slow transit constipation. When they do, straining is necessary to push out hard, rabbity pellets or thin ribbons of faeces. Because bowel contents stay inside the sufferer for longer than usual, increased amounts of fluid are re-absorbed from them. This makes the faeces harder in consistency. They may scratch the anal margin during defecation and cause blood-staining on the toilet paper after voiding.

Chronic constipation and straining at stool can lead to a number of other problems, including haemorrhoids, diverticular disease, anal fissure, and rectal prolapse.

Haemorrhoids (Piles)

Haemorrhoids are dilated, varicose veins in the rectum and around the anus caused when valves in the veins give way through excess pressure. Haemorrhoids can cause dragging sensations, itching and bright red bleeding which is sometimes copious. If large, they may cause a physical obstruction to defecation. External piles sometimes become hard, intensely painful and dark purple-black if the blood trapped inside clots. This will resolve spontaneously over two to three weeks, but consulting a doctor who will anaesthetize the area and gently evacuate the clot through a small incision brings instant relief. Use glycerol suppositories to ease motions and reduce straining. Straining can also be reduced by leaning forwards from the hips when passing a bowel motion. Drink plenty of fluids. Over-the-counter preparations (creams and suppositories) are also available to relieve the pain and itching and to numb the area. Ask your pharmacist for advice on which would suit your symptoms best. It is also important to keep the area scrupulously clean – wash with unscented soap after each bowel motion and pat dry with a soft tissue – if necessary, keep dry using a hair-dryer set on gentle heat. A doctor can treat haemorrhoids by shrinking them (by injection), tying them off with rubber bands (so they eventually drop off) or removing them surgically.

Diverticular Disease

Diverticular disease causes outpouchings of the colon wall where the mucous lining herniates through the outer muscle layers of the bowel. Diverticulae interfere with normal bowel contraction and function and may make constipation worse. Faeces may become trapped in the pouches and produce inflammation (diverticulitis) which needs treatment with antibiotics. A high-fibre diet, plenty of fluids and using laxatives to ease straining will help.

Anal Fissure

Large, hard motions can tear the anal margin as they pass through – especially if the bowel action is rapid and violent. An anal fissure is intensely painful and causes spasm that makes symptoms of IBS and constipation worse. Your doctor may recommend a local anaesthetic cream to numb the area. If healing does not occur within a few days, a chronic fissure sometimes needs a simple treatment under general anaesthetic – the surgeon simply inserts several fingers into the anus and stretches the anal margin to overcome spasm. This is known as a Lord's stretch and works by temporarily paralysing the anal muscles so that they can heal.

Rectal Prolapse

In extreme cases, constipation and straining may push an inch or two of the rectal lining (mucosa) out through the anus, where it resembles a large, moist strawberry. This can usually be gently coaxed back into the rectum by a doctor using a lubricant and local anaesthetic. If recurrent, the prolapsing mucosa will need to be stitched back in place, or excised.

A dramatic new treatment for constipation is proving successful in some hospitals. Patients are taught how to relax their pelvic floor muscles through electrodes placed on the anus. This lets the electrical activity generated through contracting and relaxing the muscles to be observed and used to co-ordinate and retrain bowel habit. On average, between three and six out-patient sessions are all that is needed. Over half the patients showed a good improvement, with a significant increase in bowel frequency lasting throughout the one-year follow-up period.

In a separate treatment advance, doctors have developed a way to retrain bowel habit using small balloons that are inflated in the rectum using a syringe. The patient performs a series of breathing and co-ordination exercises to relearn how to use pelvic floor muscles correctly. Just two to three hours' worth of treatment spread over several weeks have helped many people suffering from intractable constipation for as long as 10 years.

Causes of Constipation
Lots of things other than IBS can bring on constipation, including:

- poor fibre intake
- poor fluid intake
- weight loss diets
- diverticular disease
- inflammatory bowel disease (such as Crohn's, colitis)
- lack of exercise
- poor muscle tone
- poor toilet habit (putting off going due to being busy)
- pregnancy
- hernia
- anal pain due to fissure or piles
- depression
- old age
- prostate problems
- drugs and medications (especially opiate painkillers and anti-cholinergic agents)

- underactive thyroid gland (hypothyroidism)
- high blood levels of calcium (rare)
- high blood levels of potassium (uncommon)
- abdominal mass pressing on bowel (such as tumour, fibroid)
- disorders of the central nervous system such as MS
- bowel obstruction such as stricture due to scar tissue or colon cancer
- developmental disorders of the gut (uncommon).

DRUGS THAT CAN CAUSE CONSTIPATION

- painkillers (especially codeine phosphate)
- antacids – especially aluminium-based ones
- tricyclic antidepressants (such as amitriptyline)
- calcium antagonists (such as nifedipine)
- iron preparations
- steroids
- overuse of laxatives – so that the bowel becomes less responsive to their action
- abuse of illegal drugs.

TOXINS THAT HAVE BEEN FOUND IN A SEVERELY CONSTIPATED COLON

- phenol
- cadaverin
- agamatine
- indol
- cresol
- butyric acid
- botulin
- putrescin
- urobilin
- histidine
- ammonia
- muscarine
- methylmercaptan
- indican

- methylgandinin
- idoethylamine
- sulpherroglobine
- ptomarropine
- pentamethyl lendiamine
- neurin
- sepsin

People with constipation often complain of other symptoms, including: headache, fatigue and lack of energy, poor concentration, loss of appetite, indigestion or heartburn, coating on the tongue, bad taste in the mouth, bloating, wind, sallow, sensitive skin prone to spots.

Diarrhoea

Diarrhoea is usually defined as a loose consistency of stool plus increased frequency of bowel motions, which lasts longer than two weeks. Your doctor will want to know:

- how long you've had it
- whether the stools are watery or just soft
- if they're sloppy or like porridge
- if there are any formed stools
- their colour
- if you have noticed any blood, pus or slime mixed in with them
- whether you have feelings of urgency to open your bowels
- whether there is any sensation of incomplete evacuation
- whether you have to get up at night to evacuate your bowel
- whether the motions float or are difficult to flush away.

IBS is probably the commonest cause of persistent diarrhoea. It occurs when the bowel works overtime, to secrete increased amounts of mucus and to hasten the intestinal contents through. The problem is usually intermittent in nature and associated with other classic symptoms such as distension, bloating, excess wind and sensations of incomplete bowel movement. The diarrhoea associated with IBS is often worse in the early hours of the morning between 5 and 10 a.m. In this case, an anti-diarrhoeal drug such as loperamide will help if taken last thing at night and after the first bowel action every morning. Treatment should only be used for short periods of time, however, unless you have consulted your doctor first. It's also worth avoiding fruit juices and prunes and cutting down on milk and dairy products if your bowels are very loose. Drink plenty of fluids to counter dehydration, especially if urine production has slowed down and you are only passing small amounts of dark urine. See Chapter 10 for further advice.

Other conditions can also cause diarrhoea, including:

- bacterial, viral, yeast or protozoon infections
- overuse of laxatives
- anxiety or stress
- taking antibiotics
- inflammatory bowel disease such as Crohn's or ulcerative colitis.

Diarrhoea that lasts longer than two weeks should always be investigated to find its cause. Severe diarrhoea is debilitating and can even be fatal – especially in infants. Large amounts of salts such as sodium and potassium as well as water can be washed out through the bowels, causing dehydration, low blood pressure and shock.

Urgency

Urgency is the sudden need to rush to the toilet to open your bowels. This may herald a bout of diarrhoea, or an attack of rectal spasm and pain. Some sufferers, especially those with functional diarrhoea syndrome (*see page 28*) are unable to travel far from home because of the rapidity which they need to open their bowels. This symptom is usually made worse by following a high-fibre diet, but may respond to treatment with anti-diarrhoeal drugs.

Incomplete Bowel Emptying

Many sufferers notice an unpleasant sensation of not completely evacuating the bowels after voiding. This seems to be due to over-sensitivity of the rectum to stretching so that it continues to feel as if there is unfinished business to attend to. This may keep you on the toilet for long periods of time, and may encourage you to strain. Straining can lead to unpleasant rectal spasm (tenesmus) and rectal pain that can take your breath away and make you feel faint (*see proctalgia fugax, page 41*). If either of these two problems occurs, tell your doctor as soon as possible. You can reduce the pressure of straining by rocking forward on your hips so that you are leaning over your knees while sitting on the toilet.

Mucus Production

Increased production of mucus is triggered by mechanical stimulation of the mucus glands in the lining of the colon. It is mainly associated with the spastic colon form of IBS in which disordered contraction and motility in the colon keeps bulky, dry faeces in contact with the bowel wall for longer than normal. Occasionally, excess mucus production is a sign of a mucus-producing polyp, inflammation or infection. If mucus production is a new symptom for you, and one your doctor doesn't know about, tell him or her during your next consultation.

Nausea

Nausea is not experienced by all patients with IBS. It seems to be linked with spasm of the small intestine rather than the large bowel, and may occur in the primary foregut motility disorder variant of IBS. It may be brought on by backward passage of wind (reflux) through the intestines. If you suffer from recurrent nausea or vomiting, you should always tell your doctor.

Rectal Pain – Proctalgia Fugax (Rectal Angina)

Rectal pain, also known as rectal angina or proctalgia fugax, is a severe cramping pain, felt deep in the rectum, that is not associated with any particular condition. Most people experience it at least once in their life, including IBS sufferers, and it can be extremely frightening. It is due to muscle spasm and cramping in the rectum and may make you feel nauseated or faint, or may trigger over-breathing (hyperventilation). The pain can come on at any time – often at night – and is sometimes brought on by straining, constipation or passing wind. The spasm tends to last one or two minutes and then subsides on its own. Occasionally, it may last as long as an hour. The next bowel motion passed may take the form of a thin ribbon through having been squeezed and compressed by the cramping lower bowel and rectum. All examinations are normal and the cause is unknown. Most researchers believe it is due to spasm of the pelvic floor muscles. If you do experience a severe pain in the rectum, it is important to tell your doctor, especially if the problem is recurrent – don't make the diagnosis of proctalgia fugax yourself.

CONSULTERS VERSUS NON-CONSULTERS

Not everyone with symptoms of IBS consults a doctor. One study asked 1,058 women and 838 men – chosen at random – about bowel symptoms. The study found that:

- one or more symptoms of IBS occurred frequently in 47 per cent of women
- one or more symptoms of IBS occurred frequently in 27 per cent of men
- diagnosable IBS (three or more symptoms) was present in 13 per cent of women
- diagnosable IBS (three or more symptoms) was present in 5 per cent of men
- only half the people with diagnosable IBS had consulted a physician about it

- the likelihood of consulting a doctor was linked to the number of symptoms
- this likelihood was similar in men and women
- abdominal pain was the symptom most likely to prompt a consultation
- recurrent abdominal pain occurred in 20 per cent of women and 10 per cent of men.

If you suffer from recurrent abdominal pain, diarrhoea, constipation or other problems, it is important to seek medical advice. IBS is not a condition that you should diagnose yourself, as the bowel can only complain about illness in a limited number of ways. This means that other, treatable and potentially more serious problems such as inflammatory bowel disease, partial bowel obstruction or even a bowel tumour may be overlooked if you just dismiss your symptoms. Similarly, never be afraid to go back to your doctor with the same complaint if it does not seem to be getting better – or is getting worse. One of the skills of general practice is 'waiting and seeing' how things turn out. Self-limiting conditions will disappear on their own – those needing further investigation and treatment will be brought back to the surgery for further help.

How your symptoms can help your doctor diagnose bowel problems

Symptoms	IBS	Bowel Cancer	Inflammatory Bowel Disease
Long history of symptoms	YES	NO	NO
Spasmodic pain	YES	NO	POSSIBLE
Rectal bleeding	NO	YES	YES
Night-time diarrhoea	NO	POSSIBLE	POSSIBLE
Bloating	YES	NO	POSSIBLE
Weight loss	UNUSUAL	YES	YES
Joint/eye symptoms	NO	NO	POSSIBLE
Gynaecological symptoms	POSSIBLE	NO	NO
Stress-related symptoms	OFTEN	NO	NO

This is a general guide only, as different people develop different symptoms with different conditions.

Always tell a doctor as soon as possible if:

■ there is any change in your usual bowel habit
■ you notice any blood or blackness in your stools
■ you experience any unexplained weight loss
■ you are over 45 and develop bowel symptoms for the first time.

NON-COLONIC SYMPTOMS OF IBS

Many people with intestinal symptoms of irritable bowel syndrome also experience non-colonic symptoms. This may mislead doctors into diagnosing urinary, kidney, gynaecological or even orthopaedic problems in some sufferers. It is not uncommon for a woman with pelvic and abdominal pain to consult a gynaecologist over a period of time, and to end up having a hysterectomy. It is only when this major operation does not solve her problem, and the pain continues, that doctors realize her symptoms stem from the gut. This works both ways, however. Many women with a common gynaecological disorder – endometriosis – are often diagnosed as having IBS instead. As a result, there is an average delay of seven years between a woman first noticing symptoms of endometriosis and the correct diagnosis being made.

The non-colonic symptoms of IBS vary from person to person, and can include:

■ tiredness
■ lack of energy (lethargy)
■ nausea
■ heartburn
■ acid reflux into the mouth
■ mild weight loss
■ urinary frequency
■ urinary urgency
■ recurrent back pain
■ recurrent loin pain
■ painful intercourse (dyspareunia)
■ chest pain

- palpitations
- shortness of breath on exercise, and wheeziness
- hyperventilation (over-breathing).

These symptoms are common – up to 80 per cent of people with IBS also have upper gut symptoms such as indigestion or heart-burn. This may well result from disordered contraction and motility throughout the length of the gut.

Some doctors put these non-colonic symptoms of IBS down to general anxiety – especially if the person seems otherwise fit and well. This may be misguided, as the presence of these problems elsewhere in the body suggests that the root cause of IBS lies in an abnormality of nerve or muscle function that affects other organs and systems as well as the bowel. Researchers have found, for example, that some patients with IBS have a pattern of bowel pressure changes similar to those of the condition known as *chronic, idiopathic intestinal pseudo-obstruction syndrome*. In this condition, the bowel seems to stop working altogether due to malfunctioning of the nervous supply to the gut. This may mean that some people with symptoms of IBS also suffer from poor nerve function in the bowel. This idea is currently being investigated.

Research shows that IBS sufferers are more likely to develop symptoms of heartburn, indigestion (dyspepsia), flushing, palpitations, migraine and urinary symptoms throughout life. IBS sufferers are also more likely to develop asthma (bronchial hyper-responsiveness). In one study, 22.4 per cent of people with IBS had over-sensitive lung airways, compared with 12.2 per cent of those without IBS. This suggests that IBS may be linked to a smooth muscle disorder in both the lungs and gut.

All these findings indicate that IBS is only part of a spectrum of symptoms to which certain people are prone. They may have:

- a more active nervous system
- increased contractility of smooth muscles, including those in the gut
- increased levels of circulating vaso-active peptides (chemicals that cause constriction or dilation of blood vessels).

It may be that some people are born with a natural predisposition to IBS, and that it is only when they are exposed to a trigger factor that symptoms start. Researchers have found that people with IBS are more likely to have suffered from abdominal pain in childhood, for example – perhaps triggered by a viral illness. These recurrent attacks are often dismissed as growing pains and are eventually forgotten by parents. One study claims that as many as 1 in 6 older children has symptoms of IBS, which may be bad enough to restrict lifestyle. A questionnaire given to 851 school children found that 16 per cent had one or more symptoms of abdominal pain, altered bowel habit, urgency, and incomplete evacuation of the bowels. Boys and girls were affected equally.

Hope

Symptoms of IBS do seem to burn themselves out over time. According to one study, 70 per cent of sufferers were free of symptoms after five years. This is an indication that once the on/off switch has been identified, it should prove possible to design a drug that can effectively turn IBS symptoms off. Unfortunately, the tests currently available have failed to find an anatomical or physiological explanation for the underlying abnormal processes involved in IBS, although lots of promising research is underway.

Fertility

Female sufferers of IBS often worry that they may have difficulty becoming pregnant as a result of their condition – especially if they suffer from recurrent abdominal distension and abdominal pain. Assuming they have pure IBS, there is no cause for worry – IBS is not associated with infertility.

There is a gynaecological condition, endometriosis, which like IBS can cause abdominal distension and low pelvic pain. This is usually accompanied by pain during intercourse and period problems, however – although this is not always the case. Endometriosis is linked with infertility, although the exact reasons are as yet unknown. If you have IBS but also suffer from gynaecological symptoms, you may need to be investigated for possible endometriosis – consult your doctor for further information and advice.

Chapter Five

TRIGGER FACTORS

Different people find that different factors can trigger their IBS symptoms. A particular incident may bring symptoms on for the first time, or recurrent symptoms may be linked with some aspect of diet or lifestyle. Common trigger factors in people with a predisposition to IBS include:

- gastrointestinal infection
- taking antibiotics or some other drugs
- smoking cigarettes
- the menstrual cycle
- lack of sleep
- eating certain foods
- stress.

GASTROINTESTINAL INFECTION

Over 60 million travellers from Westernized countries visit less developed parts of the world each year. Surveys suggest that at least 50 per cent of travellers become unwell during this time with gastroenteritis (vomiting and diarrhoea). Those visiting India fare worst, closely followed by travellers to Egypt, Morocco, the Gambia, Tunisia and Kenya. Although many cases are mild and self-limiting, 30 per cent of sufferers become bedridden and another 40 per cent have to curtail their activities. The commonest organisms involved are the toxin-producing bacteria *E. coli*, *Campylobacter jejuni*, *Salmonella* and *Shigella*. Surprisingly, even 10 per cent of visitors to European resorts also get symptoms of bowel infection.

Symptoms of IBS often seem to come on or become worse after a bout of gastroenteritis (bowel infection). This observation was first made in the 1960s, but researchers are still unclear why this happens. The most likely explanation is that altered bacteria in the bowel lead to an imbalance that affects bowel motility in some way. It may cause inflammation which irritates nerve endings, or increases the leakiness of the bowel wall. By letting incompletely digested food particles through into the circulation, gastroenteritis may trigger a food sensitivity which lasts beyond the duration of the original infection. It may also encourage sensitivity to chemicals produced by Candida yeast cells (*see page 96*).

During 1994, 38 victims of an outbreak of Salmonella food poisoning were studied by researchers. Over the next year, almost a third (12 out of 38 – 32 per cent) went on to develop recurrent bowel symptoms consistent with IBS. Interestingly, five times as many women as men went on to develop IBS and, in most cases, these sufferers developed intermittent diarrhoea and bowel urgency – features of Functional Diarrhoea Syndrome (*see page 28*). In general, those with the worst symptoms of gastroenteritis (diarrhoea lasting more than seven days plus vomiting leading to weight loss) were more likely to develop IBS than those with milder symptoms. They were also the ones who took longer to recover their appetite, weight and energy levels.

Another study looked at 75 patients who developed gastroenteritis (from various organisms) which was bad enough for them to be admitted to hospital. Of these, 22 (29 per cent) had symptoms three months later that were consistent with IBS. Nine out of ten of these were still suffering after six months, and three quarters still had IBS problems one year later. Similarly to the first study, those with the worst symptoms (diarrhoea lasting longer, with abdominal pain and mucus in the stools) were more likely to develop IBS.

There is undoubtedly a link between bowel infection/inflammation and subsequent malfunction leading to symptoms of IBS. Symptoms that improve after a few months may be due to a temporary lactase enzyme deficiency (*see pages 83, 111*). Those lasting longer may be due to other as yet unexplained changes in bowel function.

In the second of the above studies, the researchers also assessed the psychological profile of the 75 patients admitted to hospital with gastroenteritis. They found that those who were most anxious, and who reported the most unexplained non-intestinal symptoms during their admission to hospital, were also more likely to develop IBS later, suggesting that psychological factors do increase the risk of developing IBS after a severe bowel infection. This may be linked with the known damping-down effects of stress on the immune system and the effects of stress hormones on bowel function. This in turn may slow recovery and result in a longer, more severe bout of illness (*see Stress, page 53*).

In these two studies, the risk of developing IBS did not seem to be related to whether or not antibiotics were taken to treat the original bout of gastroenteritis.

TAKING ANTIBIOTICS

Taking antibiotics disrupts the normal balance of bacteria found in the bowel by killing healthy bacteria (commensals) as well as those causing disease (pathogens). After the original infection has been dealt with, you may still be left with a bacterial imbalance as less desirable organisms – including yeasts – flourish at the expense of others. This can affect the normal process of fermentation occurring in the colon and change the amount and composition of bowel gases produced. Taking antibiotics frequently causes diarrhoea as a direct result of these artificial changes in gut bacteria.

While taking a course of antibiotics, it is worth eating live (unpasteurized) bio-yoghurt containing organisms such as *Lactobacillus acidophilus* or a drink (sold as Yakult) containing *Lactobacillus casei* Shirota, formulated by scientists to help re-colonize the bowel with beneficial bacteria. Many IBS sufferers claim that 'live' yoghurt every day helps to keep their symptoms under control – whether they have recently taken antibiotics or not.

TAKING CERTAIN DRUGS

As well as antibiotics, many other drugs can also affect bowel function. These include:

- laxatives
- aspirin-like drugs (such as salicylic acid, ibuprofen)
- opiate painkillers (especially opiates such as codeine phosphate and morphine)
- antacids – especially aluminium-based ones
- acid-reducing drugs – especially H2 antagonists such as cimetidine
- beta-blockers (such as propranolol, atenolol)
- tricyclic antidepressants (such as amitriptyline)
- calcium antagonists (such as nifedipine)
- iron preparations
- steroids
- hormonal methods of contraception
- sleeping tablets
- most illegal drugs
- alcohol
- nicotine.

These drugs can alter bowel motility – speeding it up or slowing it down – affect gastrointestinal secretions, disrupt mucus production, affect bowel bacteria or have a direct irritant effect on the bowel wall. If you suffer from IBS, it is wise to avoid taking all but the most necessary medications.

SMOKING CIGARETTES

Some of the nerve ganglia supplying the bowel (sympathetic ganglia) contain a type of chemical receptor that responds to a neurotransmitter (nerve chemical) called acetylcholine. These ganglia can also be stimulated by nicotine and are known as nicotinic receptors. Exposure to nicotine causes an initial burst of electrical activity at these receptor sites and then blocks them temporarily so that their activity becomes below-normal. This interferes with normal bowel function and the contraction of smooth muscle cells in the gut wall. Many people with IBS find that exposure to cigarette smoke – even passively – can cause flushing, intestinal cramps, nausea and diarrhoea. If exposure is prolonged, it may lead to constipation. It is therefore worth stopping smoking and avoiding smoke-laden atmospheres if you suffer from symptoms of IBS.

THE MENSTRUAL CYCLE

Although IBS is now known to affect just as many men as women, there are differences in bowel function between the sexes that may be linked to reproductive hormones:

- Bloating is more common in women than men.
- Bowel transit time (the time it takes for food to pass through the gut) is slower in women, especially during the second half of their menstrual cycle.
- Women excrete less bile acid than men and may digest their food less well.

Researchers have now found receptors for the two main female sex hormones, oestrogen and progesterone, in the smooth muscle cells lining the small intestines and colon. These receptors seem to be present in similar numbers to those present in breast tissue, and it is likely that they are there for a purpose. It may well be that sex hormones help to regulate gut function. During the second half of the menstrual cycle, for example, when progesterone levels are naturally high, the time taken for food to pass through the gut may be almost twice as long as during the first half of the menstrual cycle.

Oestrogen is known to have an effect on smooth muscle cells in artery walls, helping to keep them elastic, while progesterone has a relaxant effect on smooth muscle cells lining the bowel and urinary system. This is why constipation and urinary tract infections are more common during pregnancy when progesterone levels are high. It seems reasonable to assume that these female hormones may also be linked with IBS symptoms in women. Women with constipation, for example, often find that their symptoms are significantly better just before and during a period, when progesterone levels fall. Other symptoms – such as pain due to spasm – may become worse at this stage of the menstrual cycle, however. This exacerbation of symptoms does not seem to be linked with any particular psychological trait or the mood swings associated with premenstrual syndrome.

The effects of sex hormones on bowel emptying, bile acid secretion and IBS are currently under further investigation. Another theory is that the normal bacteria present in the colon are sensitive to human sex hormones – and to plant hormones (such as phytoestrogens and isoflavones) released during the digestion of certain foods. This may change the normal fermentation processes occurring in the bowel at different times of the menstrual cycle and alter the quantity and composition of gases produced.

Yet more evidence of a role for female sex hormones comes from the fact that women are more likely to develop symptoms of IBS if they have had a hysterectomy. On average, 1 in 10 women develops problems soon afterwards. In one study comparing women who had had a hysterectomy with a similar group who had not had the operation, those who had undergone surgery were more likely to consider themselves constipated, defecate less often, strain during defecation, experience abdominal bloating, have feelings of incomplete evacuation of the bowels, pass lumpy motions, and have longer bowel transit times (the latter especially in women over the age of 50).

This study suggests that having a hysterectomy can affect the function of the colon and rectum – and may possibly trigger IBS in some women.

LACK OF SLEEP

Lack of sleep can make the symptoms of IBS significantly worse. Research suggests that the severity of morning symptoms is closely linked to the quality of sleep the night before. Poor sleep may affect gut motility through an imbalance or overproduction of neuroactive hormones in the brain such as melatonin, ACTH and adrenaline. Lack of sleep also causes physical and emotional stress, with raised stress hormones (such as adrenaline) which all have effects on the gut. (*For tips on how to get a better night's sleep, see IBS and Stress, page 71.*)

EATING CERTAIN FOODS

There is no doubt that eating certain foods seems to trigger symptoms of IBS in most sufferers. For further information, see Chapter 10.

STRESS

Stress has long been known to make the symptoms of IBS worse, although there is little evidence that it can cause IBS in the first place. As one sufferer puts it, 'The only stress in my life comes from having IBS – without it, my life would be stress-free.'

Stress may make symptoms of IBS worse, but does not seem to cause them in the first place. During the stress response, the body releases powerful chemicals (such as adrenaline, neuropeptide Y, somatostatin) which have an effect on bowel function – one of the classic responses to stress, for example, is rapid bowel emptying (diarrhoea), designed to make primitive man lighter when running away from dangerous predators.

Early research found that blood flow to the colon wall increased during stressful situations and emotional arousal – so that the colon wall looked more red – and that the amount of secretions increased, as did bowel motility. These were normal responses which did not seem to trigger any unpleasant symptoms except for the expected diarrhoea.

Studies which have looked for a link between chronic stress and IBS – by examining, for example, whether nail-biting is more common in people with IBS than those without – have had varying results. In the nail-biting study, it was found that bitten nails were not a feature of IBS – but rather of youth.

Stress and the Oesophagus (Gullet)

Many people under stress feel as if they have a lump in their throat and develop difficulty in swallowing – so-called globus hystericus. It was thought that this might indicate some abnormality of muscular contraction in the upper gut (oesophagus), but it now seems that globus hystericus can be brought on in just about anyone by over-breathing (hyperventilation). This changes the ratio of gases in the lungs and affects blood acidity, which seems to interfere with muscle contraction as a normal physiological response – not due to any nerve or muscle abnormality. It is now thought that people under stress who develop this symptom have been over-breathing.

Stress and the Stomach

People under stress have increased nerve activity supplying the stomach. This can lead to increased secretion of acidic juices and sometimes churning sensations due to increased muscular activity. This is linked with symptoms of heartburn (acid reflux from the stomach up into the oesophagus) and peptic ulcers in the stomach or duodenum. There does not seem to be a link between peptic ulcers and an increased risk of IBS, however.

Stress and the Small Intestine

Studies looking at small bowel function during stress suggest that people with IBS have a more pronounced response than non-sufferers. In the normal small bowel, activity occurs in cycles depending on whether you have just eaten or have recently fasted. This pattern of activity followed by inactivity seems to be lost in some IBS sufferers under stress, so that bowel function becomes more irregular, especially during periods of fasting (such as overnight). During periods of active digestion, the number of contractions increases or decreases depending on the types of food eaten. Passage of some types of food through the small intestine is delayed, while the transit of others is increased. This is not yet fully understood, but suggests that there is an underlying abnormality in gut motility in some people with IBS.

Stress and the Large Bowel

Studies measuring electrical activity in the colon and rectum suggest that colonic activity and the number of stools passed increase during stress-testing. The ring of muscle guarding the upper part of the anus (internal anal sphincter) also becomes more constricted. These findings are not particularly linked with the development of IBS symptoms, however.

Stress and IBS

As mentioned earlier in this chapter, studies indicate that psychological factors can increase the risk of developing IBS after a severe bowel infection. This may be linked with the known damping-down effects of stress on the immune system and the effects of stress hormones on bowel function. Other researchers have found that people with IBS are more likely to have suffered from major emotional conflicts in childhood – particularly the loss of a parent, or physical abuse (especially sexual abuse). In one study, one or more of these traumatic childhood factors were found in 53 per cent of IBS sufferers, compared with 37 per cent of controls with normal bowel function. 31 per cent of IBS sufferers had been subjected to rape or incest, compared with 18 per cent of those with normal bowels.

There is no doubt that some people with IBS are also under a lot of stress or are prone to anxiety. It is worth looking at stress and how some of its symptoms can be overcome, so that if stress seems to be making your IBS worse, you can do something to help yourself.

WHAT IS STRESS?

Stress is a term used to describe the symptoms produced when you are under excessive pressure. A certain amount of stress is necessary to meet life's challenges, but too much is harmful and can leave you feeling tired, angry and tense. The symptoms of stress result from high levels of circulating adrenaline hormone which are secreted to prepare your body for conflict or escape. Adrenaline puts your systems onto red alert so that:

- Blood sugar levels rise to provide energy.
- Your bowels empty (nervous diarrhoea) so you are lighter for running – some people may also vomit if their stomach is full.
- Your pupils dilate so you can see better.
- Pulse and blood pressure increase significantly.
- You breathe more deeply (hyperventilate) so more oxygen reaches your muscles.
- The circulation to parts of the body (such as the gut) shuts down, so more blood can be diverted to muscles.

These effects were designed to help primitive man survive by fighting or fleeing from dangerous animals. Nowadays, you rarely need to fight or flee, and the effects of stress build up inside you rather than getting burned off through a sudden burst of physical activity. This means your body stays on 'red alert', leading to stress-related problems and panic attacks. Many of the physical symptoms of stress are similar to those experienced in IBS, so digestive disorders are often made worse – or attacks brought on – by stressful situations.

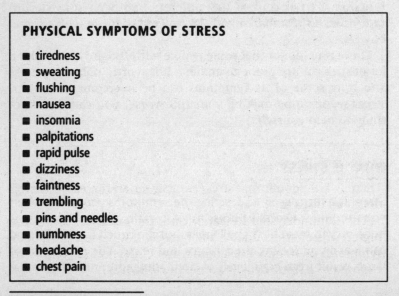

PHYSICAL SYMPTOMS OF STRESS

- tiredness
- sweating
- flushing
- nausea
- insomnia
- palpitations
- rapid pulse
- dizziness
- faintness
- trembling
- pins and needles
- numbness
- headache
- chest pain

- stomach pain
- diarrhoea
- period problems

EMOTIONAL SYMPTOMS OF STRESS

- loss of concentration
- being unable to make decisions
- a tendency to become vague and forgetful
- over-defensiveness and inability to take criticism
- extreme anger
- overwhelming feelings of anxiety and panic
- fear of rejection
- fear of failure
- feelings of guilt and shame
- negative thoughts
- moodiness
- loss of sex drive and sexual problems
- obsessive or compulsive behaviour
- feelings of isolation
- a feeling of impending doom

BEHAVIOURAL SYMPTOMS OF STRESS

- compulsive eating habits
- excessive use of alcohol or tobacco
- abuse of drugs
- avoidance of places or situations
- increased aggression
- change in sleeping habits, particularly early wakening

Stress and Illness

There is little doubt that stress can trigger an increased suscep-
tibility to disease.

The Common Cold Research Unit, for example, found that
high levels of stress double the chance of a person developing
symptoms of an upper respiratory tract infection (a cold) when
exposed to a rhinovirus (a common cold virus).

It is also known that emotional stress can worsen disease symptoms and increase your risk of high blood pressure, heart attack, stroke or even cancer.

This interaction between a person's state of mind and disease probably occurs through the immune system and may explain how some complementary therapies work. Scientists have now discovered a direct mind–body link between stress and skin disorders such as allergic (atopic) eczema and psoriasis. This link is a newly discovered protein (calcitonin gene-related peptide) that is released by nerves during stress. This substance interferes with the function of immune cells in the skin and triggers skin problems.

If you also suffer from depression, this will magnify the severity of physical symptoms associated with stress.

Personality Type

Certain personality characteristics are associated with high levels of stress: so-called Type A personalities. These people are excessively competitive, always setting deadlines and striving to get ahead. They find it difficult to relax and become frustrated and impatient with delays. They need constant reassurance of their own worth and may become hostile when thwarted. They tend to talk a lot and usually dominate conversation. They often try to finish your sentences for you and frequently look harassed and stressed. High levels of circulating stress hormones mean that physical symptoms of stress – including bowel problems – are common in this group.

Type B personalities may be equally ambitious, but lack Type A's sense of urgency. They are more self-confident and don't need to seek approval so avidly. They get on with the job and complete it to everyone's satisfaction without making a big deal about it. They are calm and pleasant to be with, easy-going, and can wait patiently to be served in a queue. Type B people can achieve just as many goals as Type A personalities and be just as ambitious, but the major difference is their lack of panic while they do so – they are much less likely to develop physical symptoms due to stress.

Whether or not you are an optimist or a pessimist is also important to your health – new research suggests that negative emotions can kill. Over 300 men and women with heart disease were assessed for personality type and classed as type-D (tendency to experience negative emotions and not to express emotions) or non type-D. They were followed for six to ten years and it was found that risk of death was nearly four times higher in those who had negative thoughts (27 per cent compared to 7 per cent) – this effect was independent of other risk factors such as blood cholesterol levels, etc.

Sources of Stress

There are two main sources of stress:

1 internal – those that come from within an individual
2 external – those that come from the environment.

Sources of internal stress include personality type, tiredness, physical unfitness, disruption of biorhythms – such as shift work, jet-lag, having to cope with a crying baby in the night – and uncertainty. Being unsure of your aims in life, feeling unable to cope with situations and a negative self-image are also potent causes of stress.

Sources of external stress are mainly related to change, particularly if change is imposed on you. Change causes uncertainty, uncertainty induces anxiety, and anxiety is a potent trigger of stress. There may be changes in relationships, in the family or at work. Above all, being unable to control situations – for example your irritable bowel symptoms – promotes feelings of frustration and inadequacy.

Life Events

Research done in 1967 by Holmes and Rahe found that an accumulation of 'life events' over a prolonged period of time greatly increased the likelihood of stress-related health problems. The questionnaire below is based on their work and will help you to consider your lifestyle and predict your risk of a stress-related illness.

Look at the list of life events below. Think back over the last two years and ring or add a tick next to any of the major life events you've experienced. At the end, add up your total score and find out how this is likely to affect your health.

MAJOR STRESS	SCORE
Death of a spouse	10
Divorce	7
Marital break up	6
Jail term	6
Death of close family member	6
Personal injury or illness	5
Marriage	5
Loss of job	5

HIGH STRESS	SCORE
Marital reconciliation	4
Change in health if family member	4
Pregnancy	4
Sex difficulties	4
Gain of new family member	4
Change to a different line of work	4
Business readjustment	4
Change in financial status	4
Death of close friend	4

MODERATE STRESS	SCORE
Increased arguments with spouse	3
Mortgage over £50,000	3
Foreclosure of mortgage or loan	3
Change in work responsibilities	3
Son or daughter leaving home	3
Trouble with in-laws	3
Outstanding personal achievement	3
Spouse begins or stops work	3
Begin or end school/college	3
Change in living conditions	3
Difficulty keeping new year's resolutions	3

Stopping smoking or drinking	3
Trouble with boss	3

LOW STRESS	SCORE
Change in work hours or conditions	2
Change of residence	2
Change in recreation	2
Change in social activities	2
Mortgage or loan less than £50,000	2
Change in sleeping habits	1
Change in eating habits	1
Holiday	1
Christmas	1
Minor troubles with the law	1
Other	add score of most similar item on list

Over the last two years, I have experienced _____ stress points.

Interpreting your Score

LESS THAN 10

You're one of the lucky ones. Life over the past two years has left you relatively unscathed. Your symptoms of IBS are unlikely to be related to stress.

11–20

Your life event score is acceptable but you need to look after your health. You've had a lot to deal with over the last two years and you may well have noticed that your symptoms of IBS play up when you are under the most stress. Take time out to pamper yourself – regular periods of relaxation are essential. Don't just sit around, follow a regular exercise programme, eat a healthy diet and go easy on the alcohol.

21–30

Your life events score is high and the stress you are under is likely to be adversely affecting your health, including triggering symptoms of IBS. Avoid caffeine and nicotine which mimic stress responses in the body and can make symptoms worse. Limit your intake of tea and coffee to three cups in total per day, or switch to de-caffeinated brands. If you smoke, try to cut down but seek help with giving up entirely – though of course this is stressful in the short term, in its own right. Vitamins C and the B complex are readily used up by the metabolism during metabolic reactions triggered by stress. Vitamin B is further depleted when alcohol and sugary foods are metabolized. Vitamin B deficiency leads to symptoms of anxiety and irritability and can trigger a vicious circle. Eat high-fibre whole foods and at least five portions of fresh fruit and vegetables per day.

OVER 30

Life has thrown so much at you over the last two years that your health is seriously at risk. Your reserves are running low and a relatively minor event may prove to be the last straw. Stressed people who have been through major life events, one after the other, are at increased risk of coronary heart disease, high blood pressure, stroke, mental illness and cancer. You should consider consulting your doctor, a complementary therapist or a counsellor about ways to help you cope with the stress in your life.

Stress Diary

Keeping a stress diary will help you to monitor the causes of stress in your life so that you can attempt to do something about them. Try to fill in your diary immediately after each stressful event – don't leave it until later or you will not remember exactly how you felt. For example:

Date	Time	Situation	Feelings	Response	Future Remedy
6/11	9.00	Overslept	Dreadful	No breakfast	Set back-up snooze alarm
6/11	9.30	Late for work	Worried	Drove too fast	
7/11	10.00	Stuck in traffic on way to meeting	Frustrated, IBS pain started	Tried classical music	Leave in plenty of time
9/11	18.00	Supermarket crowded	Hot and flustered	Rushed out forgetting to buy some things	Shop when store is more quiet

At the end of a week go back over your diary and try to iden-tify your main sources of stress and how much control you have over them. Think about your habits and consider whether any are making things worse. For example, do you always shop on a Friday evening when the supermarket is unbearable? Do you always leave things to the last minute so you run out of time?

Using your diary as a guide, try to identify:

- Are the stresses in your life internal or external?
- Are they likely to be long-term or short-term?
- How does stress make you feel?
- How does stress affect your symptoms of IBS?
- What are your preferred methods of relaxation?

Coping with Stress

Calculating average levels of stress is not possible because people react in different ways. There is no clear dividing line between stress and distress, or what level of pressure is likely to bring on your symptoms of IBS. Most high achievers, for example, would claim to be stimulated by pressure and some people appear to be addicted to adrenaline. They respond to it posi-tively and use its effects to direct their energies. However, if pressure continues at too high a level for too long, their perfor-mance will start to be affected and they may become tense, irri-table, find it difficult to concentrate, experience panic attacks or increase their reliance on alcohol and tobacco.

There are many sources of stress but they rarely exist in isolation. Few people can separate the different areas of their life so completely that home, work and play are not interlinked. Recognition of factors that cause you stress, changing what can be changed and having coping strategies ready for those that can't are the key.

Some of the solutions will be within your control, but not all. If your stress levels are moderate, the changes will be likewise. If your stress levels are high then you may have to consider drastic solutions. Stress can usually be tackled successfully by:

- changing situations that can be changed
- changing your perceptions of a stressful situation
- improving your ability to cope
- changing your behaviour
- learning relaxation skills.

Psychological Coping Techniques

The best way to cope with stress is to adapt to it in a positive, constructive manner. Situations must be seen in perspective, problems analysed logically and plans made to resolve them. As well as developing your own range of coping skills it is vital to keep fit and healthy. Make sure you don't rely too heavily on external props such as alcohol, cigarettes or drugs. These substances only mask stress and can never reduce or eliminate it – in many cases, they will also make symptoms worse by mimicking stress responses in your body.

By changing the way you look at a situation, you can reduce the amount of stress it causes. By thinking more positively, you will improve your self-esteem and self-confidence.

It is easy to compare yourself unfavourably with others. It's also very destructive. If you feel unworthy, unable to cope and inadequate, these feelings will affect the way other people look at you and they may subconsciously put you down, making your stress even worse. In contrast, if you feel happy with yourself and confident you can cope, you will feel less stressed and automatically exude an aura that affects the way other people treat you. If you catch yourself thinking a negative thought, quickly turn it into a positive one. For example:

'I can't do this' → 'I *can* deal with this problem'
'I can't cope if this happens' → 'I've coped with other problems in the past and I can cope with this one'
'This is too difficult' → 'This challenge will help me to learn new skills'

This may seem simplistic, but the power of the mind should never be underestimated. As the old saying goes, 'There's nothing either good or bad but thinking makes it so.'

Breathing Exercises

Breathing is an unconscious action which you rarely think about. Stress will quickly change your breathing pattern, so that you over-breathe or hyperventilate with quick, irregular, shallow breaths. This occurs when your fight/flight mode is triggered but not completed. As a result, you inhale too much oxygen and exhale too much carbon dioxide, causing an imbalance of gases in the lungs. This makes the blood too alkaline, leading to dizziness, faintness and the sensation of 'pins and needles' in the face and limbs. This in turn creates panic and a cycle of anxiety – hyperventilation is set up.

Fast, shallow breathing sends messages to the brain that you are under stress and keeps the body on 'red alert'. Habitual hyperventilators may also experience chest pains, palpitations, sleep disturbances and other physical symptoms. Research has suggested that chronic anxiety can be caused by hyperventilation rather than hyperventilation being a symptom of anxiety itself. Use the following exercises to control your breathing in situations where you feel stressed. They only take about two minutes each and nobody will even be able to tell you are doing them.

WHEN FEELING GENERALLY TENSE

- Sit back in your chair/car seat.
- Drop and widen your shoulders by moving your arms to draw the shoulders back and down.
- Expand your chest and take a deep breath, filling your lungs as much as possible.

- Breathe in and out as deeply as you can, being aware of the rise and fall of your abdomen – not your chest. Repeat five times. Don't hold the breath in, just breathe naturally but more deeply than usual.
- Continue to breathe regularly, getting your rhythm right by counting from 1 to 3 when breathing in and from 1 to 4 on the outbreath.

Use the following exercise when you feel panic overwhelming you. It will help you to regain control and reduce tension.

WHEN PANIC RISES

- Say 'stop' quietly to yourself.
- Breathe out deeply, then breathe in slowly.
- Hold this breath for a count of 3 and breathe out gently, letting the tension go.
- Continue to breathe regularly, imagining a candle in front of your face. As you breathe the flame should flicker but not go out.
- Continue breathing gently and consciously try to relax – let your tense muscles unwind and try to speak and move more slowly.

Stretching Exercises to Relieve Stress
Try the following when you need a quick break from your desk, or as general energizer after a long day.

ARM SWINGING

- Stand up and take a few deep breaths.
- Stretch both arms in front of you at shoulder height.
- Let your arms relax and drop to your sides, allowing them to swing to a natural standstill. Repeat several times.
- Finally, raise your arms above your shoulders and swing them energetically.

HAND SHAKING

■ Shake each hand and arm in turn for a minute or two.
■ When you stop your muscles will feel soft and relaxed.
■ Repeat using your legs and feet if you wish.

RELAXING YOUR NECK

■ Imagine you are carrying a heavy weight in each hand so that your shoulders are pulled towards the floor.
■ 'Drop' this imaginary weight and feel the tension release. Repeat several times and feel your neck become less tense.

CIRCLING YOUR SHOULDERS

■ Circle your left shoulder in a backward direction five times. Repeat with the right shoulder.
■ Circle your left shoulder in a forward direction five times. Repeat with the right shoulder.
■ Repeat, this time circling both shoulders at the same time.

Look out for signs of tension in the way you sit and stand:

CHECKING YOUR POSTURE

■ Do you stoop when sitting or standing? Concentrate on keeping your back straight, your shoulders square and your abdomen lightly pulled in – this will help you to breathe correctly using your diaphragm and abdominal muscles.
■ Do you fold your arms tightly across your chest? Try moving your upper arms away from your body and widen the angle at your elbows.
■ Do you hunch your shoulders? Try pulling your shoulders downwards towards your feet, then upwards and backwards to straighten them.
■ Do you clench your fists? Loosen your hands, so that your palms are open and your fingers curl lightly and naturally.
■ Do you clench or grind your teeth? Keep your mouth slightly open and try to relax your upper and lower jaws.

■ Do you bite your nails, twirl your hair or tap your fingers/feet? Try to eliminate these habits from your life, aiming always to keep your hands and feet relaxed.

General Relaxation

Have a bath or sit down quietly for an hour reading a book or magazine. Use an aromatherapy diffuser to fill the air with the scent of a relaxing essential oil (*see below and Chapter 9*). Have a candle-lit bath to which a diluted relaxing aromatherapy oil has been added.

Deep Relaxation

For a deep relaxation exercise which tenses and relaxes different muscle groups to relieve tension, set aside at least half an hour. This exercise is especially beneficial after a long soak in a warm bath.

Find somewhere quiet and warm to lie down. Remove your shoes and loosen any tight clothing. Close your eyes and keep them closed throughout the session.

First, lift your **forearms** into the air, bending them at the elbow. Clench your fists hard and concentrate on the tension in these muscles.

Breathe in deeply and slowly. As you breathe out, start to relax and let the tension in your arms drain away. Release your clenched fists and lower your arms gently down beside you. Feel the tension flow out of them until your fingers start to tingle. Your arms may start to feel like they don't belong to you. Keep breathing gently and slowly.

Now tense your **shoulders and neck**, shrugging your shoulders up as high as you can. Feel the tension in your head, shoulders, neck and chest. Hold it for a moment. Then, slowly, let the tension flow away. Breathe gently and slowly as the tension flows away.

Now lift your **head** up and push it forwards. Feel the tension in your neck. Tighten all your **facial muscles**. Clench your teeth, frown and screw up your eyes. Feel the tension in your face, the tightness in your skin and jaw, the wrinkles on your brow. Hold this tension for a few seconds, then start to relax. Let go gradually, concentrating on each set of muscles as they relax. A feeling of warmth will spread across your head as the tension is released. Your head will feel heavy and very relaxed.

Continue in this way, working next on your **back** muscles (providing you don't have a back problem) by pulling your shoulders and head backwards and arching your back upwards. Hold this for a few moments before letting your weight sink comfortably down as you relax. Check your arms, head and neck are still relaxed too.

Pull in your **abdomen** as tightly as you can. Then, as you breathe out, slowly release and feel the tension drain away. Now blow out your stomach as if tensing against a blow. Hold this tension for a few moments, then slowly relax.

Make sure tension has not crept back into parts of your body you have already relaxed. Your upper body should feel heavy, calm and relaxed.

Now, concentrate on your **legs**. Pull your **toes** up towards you and feel the tightness down the front of your legs. Push your toes away from you and feel the tightness spread up your legs. Hold this for a few moments, then lift your legs into the air, either together or one at a time. Hold for a few moments and then lower your legs until they are at rest.

Relax your thighs, buttocks, calves and feet. Let them flop under their own weight and relax. Feel the tension flow down your legs and out through your toes. Feel your legs become heavy and relaxed. Your toes may tingle.

Your whole body should now feel very heavy and relaxed. Breathe calmly and slowly and feel all that tension drain away.

Imagine you are lying in a warm, sunny meadow with a stream bubbling gently beside you. Relax for at least 20 minutes, occasionally checking your body for tension.

In your own time bring the session to a close.

Exercise and Stress

Regular exercise such as swimming, walking, cycling or other non-competitive sport will help you to overcome stress and make you more fit to cope with life's challenges. Adrenaline has primed you for activity and, by exercising, you will help to reverse its effects, burn off the stress hormones and reset your stress responses to a lower level. Try a non-competitive sport such as swimming, brisk walking or cycling. Spend at least 30 minutes exercising, two or three times per week – and put in enough effort to feel glowing and slightly out of breath. Even if you don't have time for regular exercise sessions, try to make activity part of your everyday routine, for example:

- Walk part or all of the way to work, for example by getting off the bus one stop earlier.
- Use the stairs rather than the lift wherever possible.
- Walk briskly around your office/workplace/home.
- Do any chores, such as hoovering, vigorously.
- Swap watching television for a family bike ride or walk.

Diet and Stress

Caffeine and nicotine mimic the body's stress response and are best avoided when you are under pressure. Limit tea and coffee to three cups per day or switch to de-caffeinated brands. Take a good multi-nutrient supplement. Some vitamins and minerals such as Vitamin C and the Vitamin B complex vitamins are quickly used up during stress reactions. Vitamin B is further depleted by the metabolism of alcohol and sugary foods, often resorted to in difficult times. As Vitamin B deficiency can in itself lead to symptoms of anxiety and irritability, a vicious circle is set in place.

- Eat little and often to keep your blood sugar levels up – never skip a meal, especially breakfast.
- Eat a healthy, high-fibre diet full of whole foods.
- Eat at least five servings of fresh fruit and vegetables every day.
- Cut back on sugar, salt, saturated fats and processed or convenience foods.
- Watch your alcohol intake and try to limit yourself to a maximum of one or two alcoholic drinks per day.

TIPS TO OVERCOME STRESS

- Work out what makes you stressed and change the things that can be changed.
- Make decisions in unhurried circumstances, not under deadline pressures.

- Set realistic goals and tackle big problems one step at a time.
- Learn to be patient, to talk more slowly and to listen without interrupting.
- Be assertive – say 'No' when appropriate and mean it – don't let yourself be put-upon and overloaded with tasks.
- Put aside relaxation time every day for a quiet read, a candle-lit aromatherapy bath or just to close your eyes and rest.

Sleep

Stress is one of the commonest causes of difficulty sleeping. Research shows that as many as one third of adults regularly have difficulty falling asleep or staying asleep.

Research also suggests that poor sleep can make symptoms of IBS worse. When 23 sufferers kept a symptom and sleep diary for a month, they found that the poorer the night's sleep, the worse their IBS symptoms next morning, with the ill effects lasting until the next evening. The researchers came to the conclusion that poor sleep may affect gut motility by causing an imbalance or overproduction of neuroactive hormones which can trigger gut spasms.

TIPS TO HELP YOU WAKE UP FEELING BETTER

- Avoid napping during the day, as this will make it more difficult to sleep at night.
- Take regular exercise, as active people tend to sleep more easily.
- Avoid strenuous exercise late in the evening, as this will keep you awake.
- Try to eat your evening meal before 7 p.m. and resist late-night snacks, especially of rich foods.
- Hunger is a primitive alerting response. The more hungry you are, the more difficult it is to fall asleep. Eat a healthy, wholefood diet with plenty of complex carbohydrates (such as cereals, bread, pasta) and fruit and vegetables for vitamins and minerals.
- Avoid overindulgence in substances that interfere with sleep, such as caffeine (coffee, tea, chocolate, colas) nicotine

and alcohol – although alcohol may help you fall asleep, you are likely to have a disturbed sleep once the drugged effect has worn off.

■ Take time to unwind from the stresses of the day before going to bed – read a book, listen to soothing music or have a bath. Add relaxing (diluted) essential oils such as *lavender, mandarin, lemon* (2 drops only) or *camomile* to the bath – or sprinkle a few drops on your pillow.

■ A warm, milky drink just before going to bed will help you to relax – hot milk with cinnamon or nutmeg is better than chocolate drinks, which contain some caffeine.

■ Don't drink too much fluid in the evening – a full bladder is guaranteed to disturb your rest.

■ Get into the habit of going to bed at a regular time each night and getting up at the same time each morning.

■ Set a bed-time routine such as brushing your teeth, having a wash and setting the alarm clock, to put you in the mood for sleep.

■ Make sure your bed is comfortable, and your bedroom warm, dark and quiet – noise and excessive cold or heat will keep you awake. A temperature of 18 – 24°C is ideal.

■ If you can't sleep, don't lie there tossing and turning. Get up and read or watch the television for a while. If you are worried about something, write down all the things on your mind and promise yourself you will deal with them when you are feeling more refreshed. When you feel sleepy, go back to bed and try again. If sleep does not come within 15 minutes, get up and repeat this process.

■ Preserve your bedroom as a place for sleep (and sex) – don't use it for eating, working or watching television.

■ Try a homoeopathic remedy:

■ If your mind is overactive: Coffea 6c

■ For sleeplessness that leaves you irritable and unrefreshed: Nux vomica 6c

■ If you are overtired and can't get comfortable: Arnica 6c

■ Take the necessary remedy half an hour before going to bed, repeating every half hour if necessary. (For more about homoeopathic treatments, see Chapter 9.)

Herbs to Help You Sleep

Some herbs have useful sedative effects to promote a good night's sleep without unwanted side-effects. Do not take a supplement containing these herbs, however, if you are using prescribed sleeping tablets, suffer from marked depression or are pregnant or breastfeeding. They may cause mild drowsiness which will affect your ability to drive or operate machinery.

PASSIFLORA

The passion flower, *Passiflora incarnata*, is one of the most beautiful and complex blooms known to have medicinal qualities. It contains compounds known as flavonoids that have a sedative and analgesic effect to reduce stress and encourage a natural, restful sleep. Passiflora is used for treating insomnia, anxiety, stress and nervousness.

VALERIAN

Valerian has been used since mediaeval times as a relaxant and is widely used as a sedative. Valerian has significant, positive effects on stress – and as well as relieving anxiety and tension, induces sleep, eases smooth muscle spasm and promotes calmness. It is also used to relieve cramps and intestinal colic.

LEMON BALM

Lemon balm is a healing, soothing herb with calming properties. It has a natural lemon scent and is widely used to ease digestive problems, nausea, flatulence, depression, nervous anxiety, headache and insomnia. May be used in combination with valerian and hops.

HOPS

Hops have a powerful relaxant effect on the central nervous system and are widely used to ease tension and anxiety and to overcome insomnia. They are also used to relieve restlessness, headache and indigestion – may be used in combination with lemon balm and valerian.

ST JOHN'S WORT

If your insomnia is linked with a low mood so you feel tearful and mildly depressed, treatment with St John's Wort (*Hypericum perforatum*) may help. Research involving over 5,000 patients has shown that extracts of Hypericum can lift mild depression within two weeks – the optimum effect being reached within six weeks. As well as lifting a low mood and improving concentration and alertness, Hypericum will also help you to sleep better.

Chapter Six

IBS AND DIET

Irritable bowel syndrome and constipation are virtually unheard of in developing countries where the local diet contains high quantities of fibre. Fibre helps digestion by absorbing water in the gut and bulking up the stools. This provides lubrication and also a weighty mass which the bowel wall can grip and push downwards as waves of muscular contraction (peristalsis) sweep past. Dietary fibre, therefore, helps to shorten the length of time food stays in the gut (bowel transit time) and helps to regulate bowel voiding.

WHAT IS FIBRE?

Fibre – or roughage – is a broad term used to describe those parts of plant foods which are indigestible. It is an essential part of our diet. While fibre provides little in the way of nutritional value, it aids the digestion and absorption of other foods.

Experiments show that for every 1 gram of fibre you eat, your bowel motions increase by around 5 grams in weight. This is because dietary fibre provides nutrients for bacterial growth, and much of the increased bowel motion bulk produced by a high-fibre diet is due to increased bacterial multiplication in the gut. Fibre also absorbs water and toxins from the gut, which increases stool bulk.

Fibre is an essential component of all plant cell structures. Fibre from different plants varies widely in its composition and its effects on the body. If you think about the differences in texture between tomatoes, cauliflower, potatoes, asparagus tips, sweetcorn and wild rice, it is not difficult to recognize some of the many different types of fibre. These will be modified to a certain extent if processed (milling, cooking, chewing) prior to being swallowed.

Humans lack the enzymes necessary to break fibre-rich foods down and release their energy, but gut bacteria can break down fibre and digest it by using a fermentation process. Certain animals (such as rabbits and cows) can obtain enough nutrients from bacterial fermentation of cellulose to survive by eating grass alone.

Soluble and Insoluble Fibre

Chemical analysis of dietary fibre shows there are two main types: soluble and insoluble. Soluble fibre is important in the stomach and upper intestines, where it slows down the processes of digestion and absorption. Blood sugar and fat levels therefore rise slowly, rather than rapidly, so the body can handle nutrient fluctuations more easily.

Insoluble fibre is most important in the large bowel. It bulks up the faeces, absorbs water and hastens stool excretion. In general, soluble fibre is totally broken down in the large bowel, whilst insoluble fibre is passed out in the motions.

All plant foods contain both soluble and insoluble fibre, though some sources are richer in one type than another.

New research suggests that bowel bacteria adapt to the types of fibre you eat. After a few weeks of eating a fibre-rich diet, these bacteria release more of the enzymes needed to break down different types of fibre – so if you mainly eat bran fibre or oat fibre, for example, bacterial enzymes will be able to break it down more easily. This means that the benefits of the fibre may be lost and your symptoms may return. It is therefore worth varying the types of fibre in your diet by eating as wide a range of fibre-rich foods as possible from a variety of sources.

The following list gives some common examples of foods rich in dietary fibre:

SOURCES OF SOLUBLE AND INSOLUBLE FIBRE

Classification	Plant Source	A Few Examples
SOLUBLE		
	oats	porridge, muesli
	barley	pearl barley
	rye	rye bread, crispbread
	fruit	figs, apricots, tomatoes, apples
	vegetables	carrots, potatoes, courgettes
	pulses	cannellini beans, kidney beans
INSOLUBLE		
	wheat	wholemeal bread, cereals
	maize	sweetcorn, corn bread
	rice	brown rice
	pasta	wholemeal pasta, spinach pasta
	fruit	rhubarb, blackberries, strawberries
	vegetables	cabbage, spinach, lettuce
	pulses	peas, lentils, chick peas

Breakfast Cereals that Are Rich in Fibre

Bran-containing breakfast cereals provide the highest concentration of dietary fibre, and there are many varieties available, including:

- muesli
- Bran Buds
- All Bran
- Bran Flakes
- Weetabix
- Puffed Wheat
- Shredded Wheat.

Recipe for Fibre-boost Apricot Nut Seed Muesli

Makes 700g of muesli mix, enough for 23 30g servings of approximately 110 kcals each. Serve with semi-skimmed milk, unsweetened fruit juice or low-fat fromage frais/yoghurt.

50g rolled oats
50g toasted wheatflakes
50g rye flakes
50g barley flakes
50g bran buds/flakes
25g bran
100g chopped dried apricots
50g chopped dried dates
50g chopped dried figs
25g chopped Brazil nuts
25g chopped hazelnuts
50g chopped walnuts
50g pine nuts
25g sunflower seeds
25g pumpkin seeds
25g sesame seeds

Mix together all ingredients and store in an air-tight container. Shake well before weighing out each serving, as the bran will tend to settle to the bottom. Replace bran with another cereal if bran tends to make your IBS symptoms worse.

FIBRE AND IBS

If you don't eat enough fibre, reabsorption of nutrients and fluid from bowel motions results in very little bulk reaching the lower colon for propulsion towards the rectum. Instead of the small muscular contractions needed to move bulky stools downwards, the colon walls have to squeeze tightly to propel the smaller pellets on their way. This is thought to lead to prolonged muscle spasm and the pain associated with some cases of IBS. As the bowel is in spasm, any additional emotional or physical stress will prolong the symptoms and aggravate the pain, as receptors in the bowel wall are sensitive to stress hormones released as a result of pain. The lack of bulk can in turn produce diarrhoea (not enough fibre to absorb excess fluid) or small, hard, pellet-like stools (because the bowel contents have stayed in contact with the bowel walls longer than usual so that more fluid is re-absorbed).

There is no consistent link between a sufferer's symptoms of IBS and fibre intake, however, and it is unlikely that a single dietary factor such as lack of fibre is the sole cause. Increasing fibre intake to 30g per day will usually help to relieve constipation (especially in patients with the spastic colon syndrome) but is unlikely to relieve wind or abdominal bloating – and may even make it worse initially.

Overall, following a high-fibre diet helps around one third of people with IBS. In up to a quarter of sufferers, changing to a high-fibre diet initially makes the bloating and distension of IBS worse. This effect disappears after two or three weeks, so it's worth trying to persevere and to build up your fibre intake slowly so your bowel has time to get used to it. In one study of 100 patients, 55 per cent said bran made their symptoms worse, 35 per cent reported no change, while 10 per cent said bran helped. Of those whose symptoms worsened, 67 per cent rated their deterioration as substantial, while 33 per cent said it was moderate.

If you cannot tolerate bran – and at least half of IBS sufferers can't – taking supplements containing other forms of fibre, such as ispaghula, psyllium or sterculia, is often effective.

Over-the-counter bulking agents come in the form of granules which are taken once or twice a day with plenty of water. The fibre swells up in the bowel and provides bulk for the intestines to grip. This helps to propel waste through the gut with greater efficiency.

Some problems related to following a high-fibre diet are due to not drinking enough fluids. Fibre in the bowel absorbs large quantities of water and can dry the gut out if fluid intake is not increased as well.

The Hay Diet

Food combining – also known as the Hay diet – has helped many people with IBS overcome their symptoms. The eating regime is scorned by many food scientists as there is no obvious theory as to how or why it works. It is essentially a healthy, wholefood way of eating that increases your fibre intake by concentrating on vegetables, fruit and salads. As it has helped so many people with IBS, it may be worth trying if your own symptoms are proving troublesome.

The Hay diet has five basic rules:

1 Fruit, vegetables and salads should make up most of your energy intake.
2 Only eat carbohydrates (starches and sugars) in small amounts.
3 When eating carbohydrates, only eat complex, unrefined carbohydrates such as wholegrains. Eliminate all refined, processed foods, additives and preservatives.
4 Don't eat carbohydrates and proteins or fruit acids at the same meal.
5 Allow at least four hours between eating meals of different types.

Books explaining the diet in depth and giving sample menu plans are widely available.

IBS AND FOOD INTOLERANCE

IBS sufferers whose symptoms are linked to particular foods often feel that some sort of food allergy or sensitivity is involved. This is a controversial area, although many researchers are starting to believe that food intolerance is linked with several common, long-term (chronic) problems such as pre-menstrual syndrome, chronic fatigue syndrome (ME), asthma, eczema, arthritis and inflammatory bowel diseases.

Food intolerance is defined as a reproducible, adverse reaction to a specific food or ingredient which occurs even when the food is eaten in a disguised form. It is relatively common. In contrast, a food allergy is a relatively rare form of food intolerance in which an abnormal immune response triggers a potentially devastating chain of reactions in the body, often involving the production of histamine and a form of antibody called IgE.

There are several medically accepted types of food intolerance and allergy, including:

- severe anaphylactic reaction – with life-threatening symptoms (falling blood pressure, difficulty breathing, tissue swelling) triggered by foods such as peanuts
- hypersensitivity – with widespread, itchy rash (urticaria), eczema, asthma, vomiting, abdominal pains or diarrhoea when eating foods such as strawberries, eggs or shellfish
- food sensitivity – chemicals in chocolate, cheese or red wine can, for example, trigger migraine
- lactose intolerance – due to an inability to digest lactose sugar in milk, causing bloating, abdominal pain and diarrhoea
- gluten intolerance – causing bloating, abdominal pain, bulky stools, malabsorption and weight loss in coeliac disease.

The type of food reaction linked with IBS is different from these and in many ways is not really an allergy at all, but a type of food intolerance which some researchers have labelled immuno-antagonism. The area is controversial, but the theory goes as follows:

When food is eaten, it is broken down in the intestines into small building blocks (proteins to amino acids, fats to fatty acids, and carbohydrates to simple sugars) before being absorbed. In some cases, however, it is thought that certain foods, to which your immune system is sensitive, make your intestinal wall porous. This is because reactive cells found in the gut lining (mast cells) burst open to attack the food with a cocktail of toxic chemicals. This causes microscopic inflammation in the wall of the gut so that cells swell and move apart, including those in the small blood vessels (capillaries), letting incompletely digested food particles enter your bloodstream. This theory is supported by research in which proteins from egg yolk and cows' milk have been found in human breastmilk. The only logical way in which they could have got there was through the bloodstream. Another possibility is that an overgrowth of Candida yeast cells damages the bowel lining as it grows through layers of cells, making the gut wall more leaky.

Once in your circulation, food particles to which you are sensitive are quickly attacked by the immune system, coated by immune proteins (complement) and destroyed by white blood cells called neutrophils. If you eat too many of the foods to which you are sensitive, however, it is thought that your immune system becomes swamped. You run out of complement proteins, and incompletely coated food particles are free to roam around your body. This challenge to the immune system has been linked with feelings of being tired all the time. The food particles are eventually filtered out in the kidneys and destroyed, but may set up mild inflammation in parts of the body linked with the chronic illnesses mentioned above. At present, this is just a theory and there is no firm evidence to confirm it, although much research continues in the area.

In irritable bowel syndrome, the increased leakiness of the bowel is thought to interfere with its function. There may also be an increase in the level of some hormone-like inflammatory agents (prostaglandins type PGE2) in the rectum which contribute to the problem. In some cases, the walls of the colon may become mildly inflamed, swollen and droop a little so that they touch and irritate sensitive muscles near the anus. These muscles interpret the stimulus as a bowel motion ready to be evacuated, and repetitive straining (tenesmus) can occur as the bowel tries to evacuate its own floppy walls. This spasm sets up a signal loop that stimulates other parts of the intestines to go into spasm and a vicious cycle is set in place, leading to spasmodic pain, diarrhoea and intermittent constipation.

Although this all remains theory at present, there is no doubt that many sufferers have symptoms that come on only when certain foods have been eaten. Researchers have found that the people most likely to have a food sensitivity and whose symptoms will respond to avoiding certain foods are those with diarrhoea.

IBS and Lactose Intolerance

Milk contains special milk proteins such as casein and a milk sugar, lactose, which can trigger intolerance in some people. Milk protein allergy is mainly found in children and is linked to diarrhoea and eczema. Most grow out of it, and it is unusual to find milk protein sensitivity in adults, even in those suffering from IBS.

Lactose intolerance, however, is relatively common and is due to a metabolic deficiency of an enzyme, lactase, needed to digest lactose before it can be absorbed. Lactase enzyme is released from the lining of the small intestine and acts on a molecule of lactose to break it down into two sugars: glucose and galactose, which are immediately absorbed into the bloodstream. Lactase deficiency leads to symptoms which can include bloating and wind, audible bowel sounds (borborygmi), abdominal pain and diarrhoea – symptoms similar to those of IBS, in fact.

Lactase deficiency can be present from birth (primary lactase deficiency) or can result temporarily after a bout of gastroenteritis (secondary lactase deficiency).

Lactose deficiency is sometimes diagnosed by taking a lactose tolerance test (*see page 111*). Results can be difficult to interpret, however, if sugar diabetes is present. A more reliable test is to measure breath hydrogen levels after a known amount of lactose has been eaten (*see page 112*). Alternatively, a small bowel (jejunal biopsy) can be taken which will confirm the lack of lactase enzyme (*see page 113*).

Treatment involves following a lactose elimination diet in which soya or low-lactose milk products are used in place of cows' milk products. If avoiding cows' milk products, you will need to ensure an adequate intake of vitamins A and D and the mineral calcium from alternative sources, including supplements.

Good dietary sources of calcium other than dairy milk products include:

■ calcium-enriched soya milk
■ eggs

- green leafy vegetables such as broccoli, spinach
- whitebait and tinned salmon and sardines which include soft bones
- nuts such as almonds, Brazils, hazelnuts
- seeds such as sesame, tahini
- pulses such as chickpeas, beans, lentils, soybeans and soybean products (such as Tofu)
- white and brown bread – in the UK, white and brown flour are fortified with calcium by law – but not wholemeal flour
- dried or fresh figs
- oranges
- prawns, cockles, mussels.

LACTOSE CONTENT OF DIFFERENT MILKS

	Lactose (g) per glass
Full fat cows' milk	9.3g
Skimmed cows' milk	9.8g
Low-lactose cows' milk	0.5g
Goats' milk	8.6g
Sheep milk	9.9g
Soya milk	0

NB: Yoghurt made from cows' milk has a low lactose content as bacterial fermentation breaks the lactose down.

IBS and Gluten Intolerance

Gluten is a protein found in several cereals including wheat, rye, barley and oats. Gluten sensitivity causes a condition known as coeliac disease (gluten sensitive enteropathy), which can come on at any age. It is relatively common, affecting around 1 person in every 2,000 – in Ireland, the incidence is 1 person in 300. It often runs in families and, classically, sufferers are said to be blonde and blue-eyed, but this is not always the case. In adults, the condition is commonly diagnosed in the third to fourth decade and affects more females than males. If symptoms develop in childhood, the sufferer is often shorter than expected due to poor absorption of nutrients from the gut.

Symptoms of coeliac disease vary. Some sufferers develop few problems and are unaware of their condition. Other sufferers develop a variety of symptoms which can creep up over months or years, and can include:

- tiredness
- generalized feelings of being unwell
- breathlessness
- abdominal pain
- bloating and wind
- diarrhoea
- vomiting
- passing pale, bulky, offensive, fatty stools that float (steatorrhoea)
- weight loss
- mouth ulcers and sores at the corner of the mouth
- skin changes including pigmentation, scaliness, easy bruising and a rash known as dermatitis herpetiformis.

The symptoms of coeliac disease are due to abnormal changes in the lower part of the small intestine, the jejunum. These changes are brought on by exposure to dietary gluten and resolve when the sufferer follows a gluten-free diet. The condition seems to be a hypersensitivity to gliadin, a small protein (polypeptide) in gluten. This may be a direct toxic effect or be triggered by an over-zealous immune system – possibly brought on in susceptible people by exposure to a particular virus.

A diagnosis of gluten intolerance is made by taking a biopsy of the small intestine (patients swallow a special capsule containing a small cutting device activated by remote control under X-ray), which can reveal any abnormal smoothness of the jejunal lining, in place of the normal tiny finger-like projections (villi). Signs of inflammation will probably also be present. This inflammation interferes with absorption of nutrients, and half of all patient also suffer from mild anaemia (such as due to iron and/or folic acid deficiency). The biopsy is usually repeated up to three times – once when eating gluten, when following a gluten-free diet, and when a gluten challenge test has been given to confirm the diagnosis.

Treatment is with a gluten-free diet, which produces a rapid improvement (within a few weeks). This diet must be followed for life – which may prove difficult in the long term. Sufferers can obtain gluten-free products on prescription from the doctor, and have to replace cereal-containing foods such as bread and cakes with gluten-free versions. They must also check food labels carefully to look for hidden gluten in products such as soups, stock-cubes and dessert mixes, etc. Vitamin and mineral supplements are important to guard against nutrient deficiency.

Although the majority of patients with symptoms of IBS will not have coeliac disease, the condition can be misdiagnosed as IBS. If you think there is a possibility that you have this condition, it's worth asking your doctor. You could also try following a gluten-free diet for a few weeks to see if your symptoms improve.

The following dietary guidelines are not exhaustive – contact the Coeliac Society for further advice (*see Useful Addresses*).

A GLUTEN-FREE DIET ALLOWS YOU TO EAT:

- special gluten-free bread, crispbread and pasta
- gluten-free flour: soya flour, potato flour, pea flour, rice flour
- soya bran, rice bran
- gluten-free biscuits, cakes
- gluten-free breakfast cereals
- rice, tapioca, sago, arrowroot, buckwheat, millet, maize, corn
- fresh or frozen meat, poultry, offal
- fish (fresh or frozen) that is not breaded or battered
- eggs, plain cheese (no added nuts, herbs, etc.)
- milk, cream, butter, margarine and oils
- vegetables and potatoes
- fruit and nuts
- tea, coffee, fruit juice
- sugar, jam, marmalade, honey, jelly
- herbs, spices, mustard, vinegar, salt, pepper
- wine, beer, spirits, etc.

FORBIDDEN FOODS INCLUDE:

- ordinary (gluten-containing) breads, crispbread, pasta
- wheat flour, rye flour, barley flour; pastry made from these
- wheat bran
- ordinary biscuits and cakes
- breakfast cereals containing wheat or oats
- barley, oatmeal, semolina
- meat pies, beefburgers, sausages, tinned meats
- fish in breadcrumbs, batter, fishcakes, etc.
- potato croquettes
- fruit pies
- barley water and some night-time drinks
- most stock cubes, gravy mixes, etc.

IBS and Wheat

Many IBS sufferers find their symptoms are made worse by eating wheat and wheat bran products. When wheat is eliminated from their diet, symptoms may improve. This may be due to altering the total amount of bran fibre in your diet rather than to a wheat sensitivity itself. As wheat also contains gluten, however, it is worth trying to work out if other gluten-containing foods such as rye, barley, or possibly oats bring your problem on too. If so, coeliac disease is a possibility.

Elimination Diet

The diagnosis of food intolerance and allergy can only be made with any degree of reliability when symptoms disappear during an elimination diet and reappear when the suspected food is reintroduced – even in a hidden form. This is best done under proper dietary or medical supervision. There are several degrees of an exclusion diet, ranging from:

- simple exclusion: the elimination of a single food
- multiple exclusion: elimination of several foods which have been linked with a particular health problem
- restriction diet: eating very few foods, for example nothing but a single type of meat (such as lamb), a single source of

carbohydrate (such as rice), a single fruit (such as pears) and drinking only spring, mineral or distilled water.

After following an elimination diet until symptoms have disappeared (commonly 10–21 days), the eliminated food(s) are reintroduced one by one, usually at three-day intervals, to see which triggers a recurrence. You will need to keep a careful food and symptom diary during this time.

Once suspected of causing symptoms, a food should ideally be given in a double-blind, placebo-controlled challenge, meaning that neither the doctor/nurse nor the sufferer knows when the suspected foods are being given. Food can be disguised or given in liquid form – if necessary through a stomach tube in hospital, for example, in cases where it is particularly important to diagnose a food intolerance accurately. You will also be given foods with which you have not previously had a problem, to act as a 'control'. If symptoms repeatedly occur only with the disguised suspect food, but not with the control substances, this confirms that the reaction is consistent and a food sensitivity is present.

Following an elimination diet is time-consuming, can be boring, and requires a great deal of motivation, but it also has many benefits.

Benefits of an Elimination Diet
A study that looked at the benefits of following an elimination diet found that just under half of IBS sufferers (48 per cent) gained some significant benefit. On average, they were found to be intolerant of between two and five different foods which, when avoided, helped to provide some relief from their symptoms. This would imply that you have a 1 in 2 chance of identifying a problem food and improving symptoms, although they are unlikely to go away altogether.

- Avoiding milk-derived foods helps 50 per cent of IBS sufferers.
- Cutting out wheat helps 25 per cent.
- Cutting out citrus fruits helps 15 per cent.
- Avoiding coffee helps 10 per cent.

It may be worth cutting out some foods such as gluten, corn, wheat, coffee, tea, citrus fruits, milk products, etc. for a while and then reintroducing them one at a time to see what happens. Keep a careful food and symptom diary, recording everything you eat and drink and at what time, any symptoms you develop, at what time symptoms start and how long they last, and your daily activities, stress levels, etc.

It may take a few days for a change in diet to affect your symptoms. If you feel there is a definite link with a particular food, keep re-introducing it after avoiding it for several days to confirm that the effect is consistent. If you are fairly confident there is a problem, discuss this with your doctor to ensure that avoiding this food is not going to cause a dietary deficiency. You may also benefit from a referral to a dietitian. It is important not to follow an elimination diet for longer than a week or two without professional dietary advice.

If, however, your symptoms are not significantly improved by following a restricted diet, it is important to return to eating a normal diet and to eating as wide a range of foods as possible, to guard against any nutrient deficiencies.

Now let's take a look at some of the other ways used to detect food allergies.

Food Challenge Tests
The food to which you are thought to be sensitive (as a result of, for example, an elimination diet) is given orally and your response noted. This can be helpful in establishing whether a particular food triggers symptoms such as those of IBS, though there is the risk of bringing on a severe anaphylactic allergic response (such as to peanuts). It should only be carried out under close medical supervision.

Sublingual Testing
A few drops of a solution containing the food to which you are thought to be intolerant (and which you haven't eaten recently) are placed under your tongue and your response noted. There is a possible risk of an anaphylactic reaction if you are highly sensitive to the food, and swelling of the tongue and throat may occur although this is rare. Used by some

alternative practitioners, though in many cases the test proves inconclusive.

Skin Contact Tests
These are sometimes used to investigate food allergies. A diluted extract is placed on the skin, and if a reaction occurs, allergy is said to be present. No one is sure how useful these tests are, as many false results occur.

Skin Prick Tests
A substance you are thought to be allergic to is applied to the skin and pricked in with a fine, sterile needle. Measuring the size of the resulting weal (if any) indicates how severe your reaction is – for a positive result, a visible skin reaction usually covers an area at least 1 cm square around the injection site. False results (positive and negative) are common, so results should be interpreted with caution. When performed by a specialist, the area showing the skin reaction may be biopsied, stained and examined under a microscope to look for the presence of immune cells. Skin tests in which an allergic substance is pricked into the lower levels of the skin (intradermal tests) can prove dangerous as they may trigger a severe allergic reaction.

Pulse Testing
Some researchers believe that after eating a food to which you are intolerant, your pulse rate will go up. This is not reliable as many factors affect the pulse rate, including anxiety, exercise, certain drugs and smoking cigarettes.

Hair and Nail Analysis
While this may provide useful information on vitamin and mineral deficiencies, it has no proven benefit in helping to diagnose food intolerance.

Antibody Screening
This can detect true allergy by looking for special allergy antibodies known as IgE. The technique, known as RAST (radioallergosorbent test), measures specific IgE antibody levels in response to the suspected allergen, but the test is not that

sensitive – false positives and negatives occur, so results must be interpreted with caution. Some patients with little specific IgE may have severe allergic symptoms, while someone with lots of specific IgE can have few symptoms.

The LEAP Test
A sample of blood is split and incubated with 50 or 100 food extracts for an hour and a half. All the white blood cells in the sample are then analysed to see if they have changed in size. If the white cells in a sample have changed in size by greater than 9 per cent, or if they have disintegrated, it suggests you are sensitive to that food. You can also be tested for sensitivity to 20 natural and man-made chemicals and 10 moulds. Results have proved controversial. (For more information about the LEAP programme, contact Oxford Nutritional Services on 01703 222007.)

NuTron Test
This takes food intolerance testing even further. A sample of blood is split and incubated with 92 food extracts for one hour. The neutrophils (white blood cells) in the sample are then analysed. As well as determining whether they become large, smaller or disintegrate, radio-frequency waves and direct-current testing detects other changes inside the cells (such as the formation of vacuoles, granulation) that would be missed by simply measuring cell volume. If any changes are found, you are said to be sensitive to that food. Results are controversial, however. (For more information about the NuTron Test, phone NuTron Laboratories on 01483 203555.)

Food Allergen Cellular Test (FACT)
Immune cells (including neutrophils, basophils, eosinophils) are incubated with food samples and the chemicals released by the cells are analysed to determine which foods you are sensitive to. Results are controversial. (For more information about FACT, contact the Institute of Individual Well-Being on 0171 495 7040.)

FOODS THOUGHT TO CAUSE INTOLERANCE AND WORSEN IBS IN SOME PEOPLE

- wheat, including wheat bran
- milk and dairy products such as cheese (but rarely yoghurt)
- yeast
- meat
- artificial sweeteners
- artificial additives
- chocolate
- gluten
- oats
- rye
- barley
- fatty foods
- potatoes
- citrus fruits
- tea
- coffee
- salads
- onions
- garlic
- pulses
- cabbage
- eggs

Recurrent Problems That Have Been Linked with Food Intolerance

- headache and migraine
- eczema and psoriasis
- painful, swollen joints and rheumatoid arthritis
- mood swings
- insomnia
- depression and anxiety
- tinnitus
- fluid retention and weight gain
- palpitations and breathlessness
- nasal congestion (rhinitis)
- constant fatigue

Vitamins, Minerals and Food Intolerance

Some researchers believe that food sensitivity is more likely if you are lacking in certain vitamins and minerals. This is common in the UK, where it is estimated that only 1 in 10 people obtains all the essential fatty acids, vitamins and minerals needed from the diet.

- 60 per cent do not obtain the RDA of 60 mg vitamin C
- 90 per cent do not get the RDA of 10 mg vitamin E
- Most people get less than 2 mg per day of betacarotene from their diet. The US National Cancer Institute suggests a minimum intake of 6 mg betacarotene per day (equivalent to 100 ml carrot juice) to reduce the risk of cancer
- Average intakes of vitamins B_1 and B_2 are below recommended levels, and 50 per cent of adults obtain less vitamin B_6 than is ideal.

The situation with minerals is even worse. The 1993 UK Government Food Survey showed that a large proportion of the population is at risk of gross deficiency in 8 out of 13 vitamins and minerals. Compared with the new EC Recommended Daily Amounts (RDAs), the average adult only obtains:

- 53 per cent of the RDA for zinc
- 56 per cent of the RDA for vitamin D
- 68 per cent of the RDA for iron
- 78 per cent of the RDA for magnesium.

And 40 per cent of people obtain less dietary calcium than recommended.

Another Government report confirms that the average intake of the mineral selenium has fallen dramatically from 60 mcg in 1978 to just 34 mcg in 1995. The ideal intakes are 75 mcg for men and 60 mcg for women.

Even when the lowest possible intake of a mineral – the amount necessary to prevent deficiency disease – is measured, a Government survey revealed the following results:

Proportion of Women with Intakes Below the Lower Reference Nutrient Intake (LRNI)[1]

AGE	16–18		19–50		51–64	
Nutrient	LRNI	%	LRNI	%	LRNI	%
Calcium (mg)	480	27%	400	10%	400	5%
Iron (mg)	83	3%	82	6%	8	1%
Magnesium (mg)	190	39%	150	13%	150	9%
Potassium (mg)	2000	30%	2000	27%	2000	23%

1   Dietary and Nutritional Survey of British Adults – Further Analysis MAFF. HMSO

And that's just for the lower reference nutrient intake. When you consider that optimum intakes of calcium are at least 800 mg per day, and that menstruating women ideally need at least 14 mg of iron per day, the number of women obtaining less than optimal levels of minerals is extremely worrying.

Increasing numbers of experts now believe that taking a food supplement is essential for optimal health. While diet should always come first, a supplement will act as a general safety net. Choose one that contains as many vitamins and minerals as possible at around 100 per cent of the recommended daily amount (RDA). Although there is no guarantee that this will improve your IBS symptoms, it will certainly guard against the common nutrient deficiencies and help to optimize your over-all health. It may also prevent some of the common, niggling health problems linked with mild vitamin and mineral deficiency. Common symptoms linked with deficiency of vitamins and minerals include:

■ lowered immunity
■ poor wound healing
■ scaly skin
■ brittle nails and hair
■ pre-menstrual syndrome
■ constipation
■ inflamed gums
■ nerve conduction problems

- muscle weakness
- mouth ulcers
- sore tongue
- cracked lips
- feeling tired all the time.

The recommended daily intake (RDA) for vitamins and minerals that meet the needs of 96 per cent of the population, are as follows:

VITAMIN	RDA
Vitamin A (retinol)	800 mcg
Vitamin B_1 (thiamin)	1.4 mg
Vitamin B_2 (riboflavin)	1.6 mg
Vitamin B_3 (niacin)	18 mg
Vitamin B_5 (pantothenic acid)	6 mg
Vitamin B_6 (pyridoxine)	2 mg
Vitamin B_{12} (cyanocobalamin)	1 mcg
Biotin	150 mcg
Folic Acid	200 mcg
Vitamin C	60 mg
Vitamin D	5 mcg
Vitamin E	10 mg

MINERAL	RDA
Calcium	800 mg
Iodine	150 mcg
Iron	14 mg
Magnesium	300 mg
Phosphorus	800 mg
Zinc	15 mg

Tips on How to Obtain the Maximum Nutrients from Your Diet

To get the optimum level of nutrients from food, you need to:

- Eat food as fresh as possible – preferably home or locally grown.
- Eat foods grown using organic farming methods where possible – these are usually significantly more expensive weight for weight, but not when measured by nutrients per pound.
- Eat as many raw fruits and vegetables as possible.
- Eat more wholegrains, nuts and seeds.
- Steam vegetables lightly or use only a small amount of water when boiling.
- Re-use juices from cooking vegetables in, for example, sauces, soups or gravy.
- Keep your use of processed, pre-packaged convenience foods to a minimum.

IBS AND CANDIDA

Symptoms of IBS have, in some people, been blamed on a yeast-like fungus called *Candida albicans*. Candida usually lives quite happily in and on the body. In its harmless form, it is present as simple yeast cells that grow and reproduce by putting out small buds which break off to form new cells. It is likely that everyone has Candida growing in their gut at some time during each year – if not permanently.

Candida albicans is the species of yeast most frequently grown from the bowel, followed by *C. tropicalis*, *C. parapsilosis*, *C. stellatoidea* and *C. guillermondii*, plus other closely related yeasts such as *Torulopsis glabrata*. All of these yeasts are usually kept under control and stopped from overgrowing by a variety of factors, including:

- competition for nutrients by bowel bacteria
- secretion of natural antifungal agents by bowel bacteria
- bowel enzymes and juices

- the action of antibodies secreted onto the inner gut lining
- immune cells that patrol the bowel wall.

Acting together, these different factors usually damp down Candida growth so that it lives quite happily inside you – and may even do some good. Vitamins made by yeast cells – especially the B-group and biotin – seep into your intestinal juices and are readily absorbed. If environmental conditions change, however, Candida can switch from its harmless (commensal) form to put out germ tubes (hyphae) which can invade local tissues. This usually only occurs if your natural immunity is weakened through:

- taking broad-spectrum antibiotics
- poor nutrition
- serious illness such as cancer or AIDS
- taking drugs that lower immunity such as chemotherapy, systemic corticosteroids, and immunosuppressants.

This is not always the case, however, and a number of apparently well people have been found to have symptoms linked with Candida overgrowth in the small intestine.

Symptoms

If Candida overgrows and invades the wall of the gut it can cause symptoms such as:

- sensitivity to certain foods
- flatulence
- bloating
- nausea
- vomiting bile-stained fluids
- abdominal pain
- diarrhoea – which is usually watery and explosive, without blood or mucus, and comes and goes over several weeks
- ulceration of the intestinal wall leading to bleeding (blood lost from this part of the bowel will usually be dark red/brown/black) by the time it reaches the anus.

One study reported six cases of small bowel candidiasis in adults, five of whom had no obvious underlying illness or immune problem – and only two had recently taken antibiotics. The main symptom was diarrhoea that lasted from four days to three months. As soon as a course of antifungal treatment (nystatin) was started, symptoms disappeared within three to four days.

In another study, 50 adults with recurrent diarrhoea and a variety of gastrointestinal symptoms were found to have a heavy growth of Candida albicans in their stool which was thought to be the cause of their problem.

Babies can also suffer from diarrhoea as a result of Candida infection of the small intestines. When 96 newborn babies with oral thrush were investigated, all were found to have Candida in their faeces as well. Thirty-three of these babies then developed diarrhoea. Of these, strands of actively growing yeast colonies (hyphae and mycelium) were found in their bowel motions. All got better with antifungal treatment. Six other babies developed diarrhoea but only had simple yeast cells in their stools – there were no signs of activation or overgrowth – and these did not respond to antifungal drugs. It is thought that diarrhoea in these babies may have been linked with an allergic reaction to the yeast cells rather than to an infection itself. Another study involving 24 babies with diarrhoea and positive stool cultures for Candida also reported that all got better within one to eight days of starting anti-Candida treatment (nystatin).

As mentioned earlier, many people with IBS develop symptoms for the first time after an attack of gastroenteritis (bowel infection) which disrupts bowel flora and may make it easier for Candida to overgrow. Researchers are unclear why bacterial bowel infections are linked with IBS, but a sensitivity to Candida products, or to a yeast overgrowth which somehow interferes with normal bowel function, have been suggested.

Candida and Food Sensitivity

While overgrowth of Candida in the small intestines produces obvious inflammation which can be diagnosed and treated, the presence of non-invasive (that is, harmless) Candida in the gut is now also thought to be linked with an allergic hypersensitivity reaction. Some researchers believe this can trigger symptoms of irritable bowel syndrome – especially diarrhoea – in certain people. This may occur after taking antibiotics. Where recurrent diarrhoea is linked with hypersensitivity to yeast cells on skin testing, and where Candida are cultured from bowel motions, bowel symptoms have been shown to get worse on being given Candida extracts to eat. Treatment to wipe out bowel Candida infection, plus a yeast-free diet (*see page 100*), can help.

In many cases, however, anti-Candida treatment has not improved symptoms. Rather than dismissing Candida as a cause, researchers should instead look for another explanation of how Candida may play a role in IBS. It may be that an overgrowth of Candida has damaged the bowel wall enough to make it leaky, so that other chemicals – including partially digested food particles – which do not usually reach the bloodstream are absorbed. This may set up an immune response known as immuno-antagonism (*see page 81*), in which case the presence of Candida acts as a trigger for IBS, though not causing it directly. Once the damage is done and the bowel and immune system are sensitized to these food particles, treatment to eradicate the yeast overgrowth could not be expected to help.

Investigation of Bowel Candida

Candida infection of the small bowel may be suggested by abdominal X-rays which show thickened and dilated loops of bowel. Small bowel biopsy and endoscopic examination (using an endoscope, an instrument containing a light source, lens system and room through which to pass instruments such as biopsy forceps) will show yeast infiltration of tissues.

In severe cases, endoscopy of the duodenum and upper jejunum may reveal multiple small white patches (plaques) and ulceration in the bowel wall. This leads to swelling of the bowel lining and dilation of loops of bowel.

Occasionally, it may be necessary to take a biopsy of the lower part of the jejunum (*see page 113*).

Treatment

A definite Candida infection of the intestines can be treated with antifungal drugs such as:

- Nystatin (tablets or suspension) taken four to six times daily for as long as necessary
- Fluconazole (capsules or suspension) – taken once a day for 14–30 days
- Ketoconazole – taken once a day for at least one week after symptoms have gone
- Miconazole – tablets taken four times a day for 10 days, or up to two days after symptoms have cleared
- Amphotericin – given by mouth four times daily, or as a special solution given intravenously for severe infections.

Anti-Candida Diet

While the theory remains controversial, some researchers have linked IBS symptoms with a sensitivity to Candida yeasts in the gut. Candida yeasts mostly enter your gut through your mouth:

- in the food that you eat
- from the skin of your hand when eating food or licking your fingers
- by sucking items that may have yeast cells on them
- through kissing and oral sex.

Following an anti-Candida diet is designed to reduce the chance of ingesting yeast cells, and to limit the growth of those already present in your bowel.

Live Candida yeasts are frequently present in food and drinks. In one study analysing a range of common foods, live Candida cells were recovered from a number of items.

Type of Food	Number of samples tested	Number positive for live Candida yeasts	per cent
Drinks	16	4	25 per cent
Breads	8	0	0
Cereals	17	2	12 per cent
Condiments	23	0	0
Desserts	39	1	3 per cent
Fish	4	0	0
Fruits	6	0	0
Juices	61	38	62 per cent
Meats (cooked)	20	0	0
Milk and products	27	1	4 per cent
Salads	8	3	38 per cent
Sauces	10	0	0
Snacks	25	3	12 per cent
Soups	16	0	0
Vegetables	44	2	5 per cent
Ready-cooked meals	21	0	0

With the juices, all vegetable and fruit types were affected, including apple, pineapple, orange, tomato, grape, apricot and lemonade. The yeast contamination seemed to be related to the type of packaging and processing used during preparation rather than the type of fruit involved. All juices sealed with foil wraps were contaminated, while those in cans or bottles were yeast-free.

There is no doubt that many people with IBS notice a significant improvement in their symptoms if they follow a low-yeast – so called anti-Candida – diet. This involves avoiding products containing brewer's or baker's yeast, and products that promote their growth such as refined carbohydrates and sugar.

■ Avoid refined carbohydrates (such as white flour) and products made from them, as well as generally lowering your carbohydrate intake. This goes against most healthy eating guidelines (which encourage you to eat more unrefined complex carbohydrates), so if after a few weeks you have not noticed a significant benefit from following the anti-Candida regime, it is important to return to a normal pattern of healthy eating.

- Avoid white or brown sugar and food or drinks containing these (such as honey, jam, desserts, treacle, cakes, biscuits, sauces, ice-cream, soft drinks, dried fruits, chocolates, etc.).
- Avoid products containing yeast such as yeast extracts, cheese, bread made with yeast, alcoholic drinks, vinegar and pickled foods, grapes and grape juice, unpeeled fruits, dried fruits, frozen or concentrated fruit juices, old (potentially mouldy) foods, mushrooms, and B-vitamin supplements not labelled as 'yeast-free'.
- Eat lots of foods that tend to contain natural antifungal agents such as garlic, herbs and spices, and fresh green leafy vegetables.

If you are not overweight and find you lose more than one or two pounds on the above regime, it is important seek nutritional advice from a dietitian. This can be arranged through your own doctor.

How to Boost Your Immune System

To generally boost your immune system without sticking to an anti-Candida regime:

- Follow a wholefood diet containing plenty of peeled fresh fruit, vegetables and wholegrains, with as few processed foods and additives as possible.
- Cut back on your intake of omega-6 polyunsaturated vegetable fats (found in margarines, cakes, biscuits, etc.) and eat more omega-3 essential fatty acids (such as those found in oily fish).
- Take a good vitamin and mineral supplement providing as many vitamins and minerals as possible at around 100 per cent of the recommended daily amount (RDA).
- Consider taking higher doses of the antioxidant vitamins C and E.
- Consider taking pure evening primrose oil supplements (*see page 137*).

- Check whether you are zinc deficient by obtaining a solution of zinc sulphate (5 mg/5 ml such as Lambert's DuoZinc solution) from a pharmacist. Swirl a small amount in your mouth. If it seems tasteless, you are significantly zinc deficient; if it tastes fuzzy, slightly sweet or mildly of minerals, you have a borderline zinc deficiency; if it tastes foul you are not zinc deficient. If you *are* zinc deficient, take 10 mg zinc twice per day for two weeks, then re-test using the zinc sulphate solution.
- If you smoke, stop.
- Limit your alcohol intake to no more than 1–2 units per day.
- Try eating live (unpasteurized) bio-yoghurt containing organisms such as *Lactobacillus acidophilus*, or a drink containing *Lactobacillus casei* Shirota (Yakult) to help colonize your bowel with friendly bacteria.
- Take regular exercise.
- Obtain adequate rest and sleep.

Chapter Seven

TESTS AND INVESTIGATIONS

Unfortunately, there are no positive diagnostic tests for IBS that can definitely confirm you have the condition. Because so many other bowel problems produce similar symptoms, any investigations are intended to rule out other conditions such as ulcerative colitis, Crohn's disease, diverticular disease and bowel cancer.

Originally, IBS was looked on as a diagnosis of exclusion – it was only diagnosed once other more serious bowel problems were ruled out. This view is now less common, as for most people, it would lead to many unnecessary and at times unpleasant investigations. Instead, careful questioning is used more and more to diagnose IBS on clinical grounds. This avoids unnecessary tests, while at the same time providing reassurance for both patient and doctor that an organic problem such as inflammatory bowel disease or bowel cancer has not been overlooked.

You may have some of the following investigations during evaluation of your bowel symptoms, but it is rare to have them all. As a routine, most people with symptoms suggestive of IBS are likely to have some basic blood screening tests and a sigmoidoscopy. If you are aged over 45, or have lost weight recently, you will probably have further investigations such as a barium enema or colonoscopy. If you are suffering from diarrhoea, a small biopsy of your bowel wall may be taken (such as during sigmoidoscopy) for examination to rule out inflammatory bowel disease. You may also have a lactose intolerance test and a biopsy of the small intestine if lactase deficiency is thought to be a possibility.

In pure IBS, all tests should produce normal results. Unfortunately, being told by a specialist that all the tests are negative is upsetting – until you realize that the doctor is not trying to say you are imagining your symptoms, but that nothing potentially serious or life-threatening is present. This reassurance that symptoms are due to IBS means that different treatments – drugs or self-help regimes – can be tried to see which suits you best, with no fear that another diagnosis requiring a different treatment has been missed.

ABDOMINAL EXAMINATION

Abdominal examination (palpation) is essential to look for signs of tenderness, fullness or obvious masses. Usually abdominal examination reveals nothing abnormal in IBS, although some patients will have a boggy colon (known as 'the squelch sign') and the last part of the colon (sigmoid colon) may be loaded with faeces and therefore tender. This tenderness may be found down the lower left-hand side of your abdomen (descending and sigmoid colon) or on the right (position of the ascending colon).

RECTAL EXAMINATION

A digital rectal examination is important for anyone with a bowel problem. This is only slightly uncomfortable and gives important information regarding the texture of the bowel lining and whether the rectum is full or empty of stool. It can enable the detection of rectal tumours as 75 per cent of them are within reach of the examining finger.

It is nowhere near as unpleasant as most people think, but can be uncomfortable. Most patients describe the sensation as similar to that experienced when constipated. The doctor uses a colourless, water-based jelly as a lubricant. Only the index finger is inserted – which if you think about it, is much thinner than the width of the average bowel motion.

The doctor will first inspect your anus and surrounding skin, looking for skin rashes and scratches, obvious leaking of faeces, blood or mucus, scars or unusual openings (fistulas), lumps and bumps (such as piles, warts, prolapsed piles), and ulcers, especially a fissure.

The doctor will then place the pulp of his or her index finger on the centre of your anus and gently press inwards and backwards. He or she will gently examine all around the inside of your lower rectum, feeling for and assessing the tone of your anal sphincter, the texture of the rectal walls, the contents of the rectum (usually it is empty – if there are faeces present, whether they are hard or soft; if the rectum is empty, whether it is ballooned out), any pain or tenderness, any thickening or mass, any internal ulceration, and any internal irregularity or hardness. If the patient is male, his prostate gland can also be assessed. If female, the cervix and uterus may be assessed.

You may be asked to bear downwards so the doctor can feel further up. The doctor may also press on your abdomen (bimanual examination) at the same time. On withdrawing his or her finger, the doctor will examine the glove to note the colour of the faeces, and see if any blood or mucus is present.

Don't be embarrassed if you leak fluid, faeces or wind. Doctors are used to this.

In IBS, the results of a digital rectal examination will be entirely normal, although the lining of the rectum may seem loose in some people.

BLOOD TESTS

Most people with symptoms of IBS will have routine blood tests performed to rule out problems such as anaemia (low haemoglobin), infection (high white cell count) or an underactive thyroid gland (low thyroxine [T4] with a high level of thyroid-stimulating hormone [TSH]). If you have diarrhoea, the salt balance of your body (sodium, potassium) will be measured to make sure you have not developed a low potassium level due to excessive fluid loss. Sometimes liver and kidney tests are requested routinely as a baseline. Measuring the stickiness of your blood (plasma viscosity [PV] or the erythrocyte sedimentation rate [ESR]) will indicate if any inflammatory processes are going on in your body.

If coeliac disease is suspected, it is possible to perform a special blood allergy test to detect antibodies against gliadin, the small protein (polypeptide) found in gluten, to which sufferers are sensitive. A sample of blood fluid (serum) is split, diluted, and incubated with special beads which are pre-coated with gliadin. If antibodies are present in the person's blood, they will bind to the gliadin on the beads. In the next step, the beads are washed and then exposed to fluorescent antibodies which will in turn react with any antibody previously bound to the beads. If the antibody was present in the patient's blood, the beads will then fluoresce bright green when looked at under a microscope. This test is not yet widely available and may give false positives in some patients with other illnesses involving the gut.

STOOL CULTURE

If you have prolonged or recurrent diarrhoea, your stools will usually be cultured to look for signs of infective bacteria, viruses or other parasites. This is especially important if you have recently travelled abroad, if other members of your family are affected or if your occupation involves food handling. You will need to provide a fresh stool sample which is preferably sent to the hospital while it is still steaming to increase the chances of any pathogens being found. It will take a few days for the stools to be cultured and the results to become available.

FAECAL OCCULT BLOODS

In this test, a small sample of stool is smeared onto a special reagent paper containing a chemical (such as the gum guaiac) which reacts with hidden (occult) blood and changes colour when activated by a developer. This test is a routine screen for early bowel cancer, but false positives are common – especially if you have cleaned your teeth vigorously the night before, eaten red meat or have piles. If the test comes back positive, it will be repeated two or three times before any decision to investigate further is taken.

ABDOMINAL X-RAY

An abdominal X-ray is not usually very helpful, but is sometimes requested to rule out abnormal collections of fluid or air in the abdominal cavity. It is often performed at the beginning of a barium enema to provide images for comparison with those obtained during the procedure.

ULTRASOUND

During this investigation, which is simple and painless, a special probe is run up and down the outside of your abdomen to pass high-frequency, inaudible sound waves through your body. This is the same test used during pregnancy to check the development of a growing baby. The ultrasound waves bounce back off tissue planes and collections of fluid or air to give a pattern that is interpreted by a computer to form an image. Ultrasound is best done with the patient's bladder full, to help orientate the images produced.

PROCTOSCOPY

This involves visually examining the inner walls of the rectum. A small, lubricated speculum is inserted to expose the rectal wall lining. This helps the doctor to see if the rectum is inflamed or bleeding, or has internal piles or other lesions. In pure IBS, proctoscopy will reveal nothing but perfectly normal and healthy looking tissues.

SYGMOIDOSCOPY

A sigmoidoscope is used to view the inner walls of the lower (sigmoid) part of the colon. There are two sorts of sigmoidoscope – rigid and flexible. The rigid sigmoidoscope is a narrow instrument around 30 cm long with illumination at the end. It has several channels along it through which the surgeon can pass air or a special instrument to take a biopsy. The rigid sig-moidoscope lets the doctor examine your bowel lining up to around 20 cm of the anus. The flexible sigmoidoscope can pass further up, allowing 60 cm of the lower bowel to be visually inspected using fibre-optics.

During either procedure, you will be asked to lie on your left side, with your knees drawn up slightly. After gently inserting the narrow end of the instrument into the lower rectum, air is pumped into your bowel to spread the walls gently apart, away from the advancing tip of the instrument. As this air escapes it may produces noises similar to flatus and many patients are embarrassed by it. Remember, though – it's not *your* wind caus-ing the problem, but that pumped in by the doctor. No one else in the room will think anything of it, so try not to be upset. During the procedure, the doctor will assess the appearance (colour, granularity, sheen) of the bowel lining (mucosa) and look for any obvious inflammation, bleeding sites, masses or polyps. He or she will also note how strongly and frequently your lower bowel contracts when the instrument is advanced. If contractions are powerful – known as 'the winging sign' – it is a good indication that the type of IBS associated with consti-pation, rectal distension and abdominal pain (spastic colon syn-drome) is present. It implies that your symptoms can probably be brought under control by taking measures to eliminate con-stipation and rectal distension.

The air pumped into your bowel may also cause distension pain similar to your usual IBS symptoms. If this happens, it is important to tell the doctor – again, this is a good sign that your symptoms are related to muscular activity within the bowel rather than to any other disease process.

Some of the wind pumped into your bowel may remain inside for a day or so afterwards, causing distension, discomfort and flatus, although most patients have few problems.

COLONOSCOPY

Colonoscopy uses a longer, flexible instrument than the sigmoidoscope, to inspect further up the colon, usually with the patient under light sedation. You will be given a powerful laxative (or oral bowel-cleansing solution) to take beforehand, which acts within 10 to 14 hours. This helps to empty the bowel and provide a better view for the doctor.

Colonoscopy is usually only performed if a change in bowel habit such as constipation or diarrhoea is accompanied by persistent bleeding or weight loss, or if there is a family history of bowel problems. It is more accurate than a barium enema but is limited by its poor ability to reach the first part of the colon (caecum). People aged 40–50 years are often investigated routinely (because for this age group bowel tumours have to be considered), though the percentage of abnormal findings picked up is low.

BARIUM ENEMA

Soft tissues such as the bowel do not show up very well on X-ray. One way to examine your bowel is to coat its internal lining with a substance that shows up on X-ray, such as barium sulphate. Before having a barium enema, you will be asked not to eat anything the night before, and to drink plenty of fluids instead. You will also be given a powerful laxative to empty your bowel so that faeces don't get in the way of the test.

The test will take part in the hospital radiology department. A tube is gently inserted into your rectum and a small amount of barium mixture pumped in along with some air to provide a good contrast on the X-ray. During the procedure you will be asked to lie on a special table that allows your body to be tilted up and down at different angles. This lets gravity do the work of spreading the barium solution to coat your inner bowel walls. The radiologist will watch views of your bowel the whole time, and print radiographs at certain times, especially if anything unusual such as an ulcer or solid mass shows up. While a barium enema usually provides good views of the first part of the colon (caecum), any faeces sticking to the bowel walls will interfere with the results. They can show up as solids which may be misinterpreted as a polyp or tumour requiring subsequent colonoscopy for further inspection. The overall accuracy of a barium enema is therefore usually quoted as around 85 per cent.

Having a barium enema is not the most pleasant experience in the world, as it can be uncomfortable, noisy and messy. It is not usually painful, however. Afterwards, the solution will be passed as a runny bowel motion. You may pass wind and have white, lumpy bowel motions over the next few days.

TRANSIT BOWEL STUDIES

Some people with severe constipation may be offered transit studies to see how fast bowel contents move through the gut. You will be given a special substance to swallow which gives off safe amounts of radio-isotopes or other markers that can be accurately measured. If, 96 hours later, 20 per cent or more of these markers have not been voided, and are still detectable in your gut, this shows that transit of bowel contents is sluggish.

BOWEL PRESSURE STUDIES

Abnormality of bowel contractions (motility) can be mapped out using small-diameter tubes containing pressure sensors. These are placed in the intestines to record motility changes which can be relayed to show pressure changes occurring throughout a 24-hour period.

LACTOSE TOLERANCE TESTS

In the classic test, a dose of lactose sugar (up to 100g dissolved in 400ml water) is taken by mouth. A sample of blood is taken at the beginning of the test, then at 15, 30, 60, 90 and 120 minutes later to assess blood sugar levels. These samples are usually taken through a special canula placed in a vein at the side of your wrist so that you don't have to have repeated needle stabs. Symptoms such as bowel distension, pain, flatulence and diarrhoea are also noted throughout the test. If blood sugar levels fail to rise above a certain level (less than 26mg/100ml – 20mg/100ml if capillary blood from fingerprick testing is used), then lactose digestion (breakdown to glucose and galactose) and absorption is abnormal and implies a deficiency of lactase enzyme.

Another test, the ethanol galactose test, involves giving an alcohol load (300mg ethanol/kg body weight) over 5 to 10 minutes followed by 50g lactose sugar solution. A blood sample is taken at the beginning and again after 40 minutes, and blood galactose levels are measured. A rise in blood galactose of less than 5mg/100ml is considered abnormal and implies that lactose digestion and absorption is faulty.

A more reliable test is to measure breath hydrogen levels after a known amount of a carbohydrate such as lactose is eaten. In normal conditions, the hydrogen content of the breath does not increase as all lactose is absorbed. If there is a deficiency of lactose, the sugar reaches the colon where bowel bacteria ferment it to produce an increase in breath hydrogen content after around 90 minutes of eating. You will be asked to fast overnight. Your baseline hydrogen excretion rate is measured and you are then given a dose of lactose (around 20g in solution). Using a special rebreathing technique to concentrate hydrogen gas, expired air is collected in four-minute samples. In normal people who produce enough lactase enzyme, the rise in hydrogen gas levels should be less than 0.3 ml/minute. A rise in hydrogen levels implies that unabsorbed carbohydrate has reached the colon. Taking laxatives, antibiotics or using enemas may affect the result. Smoking can also increase breath hydrogen levels and interfere with the results.

In a modification of this test, lactose labelled with a safe radio-active carbon atom is given. Air samples are then collected after one, two, three and four hours to see how much radio-active labelled carbon-dioxide gas you exhale. This test is one of the most accurate available, but it is expensive and only usually used by well-funded researchers.

Alternatively, a small bowel (jejunal) biopsy can be taken to provide a definitive answer about whether someone has lactose intolerance. The biopsy tissue is broken up and incubated in a solution containing lactose, to measure accurately how much lactase enzyme activity is present.

JEJUNAL BIOPSY

A small, cylindrical metal device (such as what is known as a Crosby capsule) is attached to 2 metres of polyethylene tubing. The tubing is filled with saline and the capsule swallowed so that the tubing trails from the mouth as the capsule progresses through the bowel. Its position is monitored by X-ray or positioned using an endoscopic viewing instrument. When the capsule is in the lower part of the small intestine (jejunum), a syringe is attached to the end of the tubing and suction used to produce a slight vacuum. This gently sucks the bowel lining up against a small hole in the capsule. This in turn activates a spring-loaded knife-blade within the capsule which snips off a tiny piece of the bowel lining. The activation of the knife can be heard as a distinct click by listening to the abdomen with a stethoscope. The capsule is then gently pulled back up through the gut to retrieve the biopsy. This test has been widely used for almost 40 years and is perfectly safe. Its drawbacks are that it is relatively time-consuming, the capsule is frequently withdrawn and found to be empty of any biopsy, or the capsule becomes detached from its tubing during withdrawal so that the patient's stools have to be collected and sieved for several days afterwards to retrieve the metal cylinder.

COMPUTED TOMOGRAPHY (CT SCAN)

A CT scan is not often performed during investigation of IBS unless there is a suggestion of a mass in the abdomen. This is because the procedure is expensive and exposes you to radiation, so is only performed where it is likely to provide some significant benefit. CT scans involve taking multiple X-ray views across your body at different angles, which are then interpreted by computer to produce a cross-sectional image (slice) at various levels.

MAGNETIC RESONANCE IMAGING (MRI)

MRI does not involve the use of X-rays and is therefore preferable to a CT scan if this type of procedure is indicated. It uses a strong magnetic field to align the molecules in your body. A pulse of radio waves is then passed through you to knock the molecules slightly out of alignment. As the molecules bounce back into place, they give out a weak radio signal which is picked up and interpreted by a computer. This gives an excellent cross-sectional or 3-D image of different parts of your body without any known risks or side-effects. It is expensive, however, and the more expensive tests are only done if absolutely necessary – that is, not routinely.

Chapter Eight

MEDICAL TREATMENT

A number of preparations are available over the counter or on prescription to help treat the symptoms of IBS. This chapter looks at some of these, giving information on possible side-effects and those for whom some drugs may not be suitable. Clinical trials involving different drugs have suggested that inactive preparations (placebos) can also be effective in as many as 40–70 per cent of cases – even when the sufferer knows the treatment is inert. Unfortunately, this has put some doctors off prescribing drugs for symptoms such as constipation and diarrhoea.

If you are taking other medicines, always check with your doctor or pharmacist, before starting a new treatment, that the drugs will not interact. Do not take any drugs if pregnant or breastfeeding, except under medical advice.

If you develop any side-effects which you think may be linked with your medication – even if not listed here as possible side-effects – always tell your doctor.

LAXATIVES

It is estimated that 14 million people in Great Britain take laxatives on a regular basis, although less than one in four of these consider themselves to have constipation. The overall effect of laxatives is to increase the fluid content of bowel motions, increase intestinal motility, and in some cases alter the way in which the colon contracts. Six out of ten users take a stimulant laxative which works by irritating the colon, which may make symptoms of IBS worse. Prolonged use will trigger insensitivity to the laxative so that more and more has to be taken to achieve the same effect – their effectiveness becomes reduced and rebound constipation can occur when the laxative is stopped. If constipation lasts more than a few days, check with your doctor before continuing using a laxative treatment.

Tips on Using Laxatives

Laxatives can help when used wisely. As a general rule:

- Do not use in the presence of undiagnosed abdominal pain, nausea or vomiting.
- Only take them when absolutely necessary and do not mix them.
- Do not use during pregnancy or when breastfeeding, except under medical advice.
- Use the mildest one to cope with your symptoms – if in doubt, consult a pharmacist.
- A bulking agent (such as fibre supplements) or gentle osmotic laxative (such as lactulose) is a good first-line agent to try.
- Stimulant laxatives such as senna should be avoided as much as possible.
- Rectal preparations (suppositories, micro-enemas) are often as helpful as – or better than – taking an oral laxative, and less likely to cause side-effects.
- Do not exceed the stated dose.
- Drink plenty of fluids and increase the amount of fibre in your diet.
- Take regular exercise.
- Try abdominal massage to encourage peristalsis and bowel emptying (*see page 131*).
- Taking a tablespoon or two of cold-pressed oils such as virgin olive oil, safflower, walnut or sesame can help to get constipated motions moving.

Laxatives fall into four main groups depending on how they work:

1 bulking agents – mild
2 faecal softeners – mild
3 osmotic agents – Lactulose is gentle; some salts have a strong action.
4 stimulants – moderate irritant action.

Bulking Agents

Bulking agents contain indigestible plant fibre that is taken with water or sprinkled onto food. They increase the volume of bowel motions by absorbing water, softening the faeces and helping the bowel walls to get a better grip for propelling motions downwards. They work very well, but it is important to drink plenty of water with them. Some people find them unpalatable, and the added fibre may cause flatulence and bloating, making IBS symptoms worse. Don't keep taking the same sort of fibre product month after month, as its effectiveness will decrease and your symptoms may return as your bowel bacteria adapt to it. Keep varying the types of fibre that you eat (*see page 76*):

- natural bran – introduce at a dose of 1 tablespoon two to three times a day with meals and vary according to response
- wheat husks
- ispaghula husks
- sterculia
- methyl cellulose.

The onset of action for bulking agents is slow and gentle: usually 12 to 24 hours, but may take several days. You will need to persist with treatment for a week or two before you establish a regular bowel pattern.

Bulking agents should not be used by people with undiagnosed abdominal pain or vomiting in case a degree of bowel obstruction is present. They are also useful for absorbing excess fluid in people with functional diarrhoea.

Faecal Softeners

Faecal softeners work by increasing the penetration of water and fats into motions. This softens them, eases straining and is useful for painful conditions such as anal fissure, haemorrhoids, proctitis, and where straining should be avoided. Onset of action: 24 to 48 hours.

Paraffin

This type of faecal softener has a lubricating action. Hardly any is absorbed from the gut and it is relatively safe, although some people find it unpleasant to take. The use of liquid paraffin should be restricted to temporary relief of constipation. Repeated use is not advised as it can affect absorption of vitamins and minerals in the gut, and may seep through the anus causing irritation and embarrassing moistness. There is a possible risk of respiratory inhalation in debilitated patients which may lead to pneumonia. Should not be taken immediately before going to bed.

Docusate Sodium

This has a detergent action to reduce the surface tension of bowel motions and encourage softening through water absorption. Also stimulates the secretion of water and salts into the gut and can be classified as a stimulant laxative, too. Treatment is usually started with larger doses (up to 50 ml per day in divided doses) which are decreased as symptoms improve. May cause an unpleasant aftertaste or burning sensation, which can be minimized by drinking plenty of water after taking the solution.

Osmotic Laxatives

Osmotic laxatives work by drawing fluid into the bowels to soften stools and provide lubrication to ease constipation. They should always be taken with plenty of water. Salts of sodium, potassium or magnesium have a powerful action and are also known as saline purges. Their onset of action is rapid – within one to four hours in some cases – and can verge on the violent or incontinent. Lactulose is one of the gentle members of this group, usually working within 24 to 48 hours after the first dose.

Lactulose/Lactitol

Lactulose is a synthetic double sugar (disaccharide) that is not digested or absorbed from the small intestine. It has an osmotic effect which draws water into the bowel and interferes with fluid absorption. Once in the large bowel, lactulose is digested by normal colonic bacteria which convert it into short-chain organic acids. This encourages bacterial growth, bulks up the size of the stool and raises stool acidity. These actions encourage peristalsis and help to move moist faeces through the colon. Available as a liquid or as a dry powder (which some people find unpalatable as it is quite sweet). Safe for use by pregnant or lactating women, the elderly, diabetics and children over the age of five.

Magnesium Salts

Magnesium salts are useful when rapid emptying of the bowel is needed (such as before a bowel investigation) and for some people with an abnormally slow bowel transit time. Should be restricted to occasional use only. May cause colic. Should not be used by those with poor kidney or liver function except under medical advice.

Sodium Salts

It is not recommended that sodium salts be taken by mouth, as they may cause salt and water retention in some people. Should not be used by people with high blood pressure, heart or kidney problems except under medical supervision. Mainly used rectally as micro-enemas.

Stimulant Laxatives

Stimulant laxatives work by irritating the bowel wall and increasing colonic motility. Some purge the bowel and can cause a sudden, violent action of watery motions with intestinal cramps and griping. This will obviously make IBS symptoms worse. They should only be used on specific occasions and are best avoided by most people with IBS. If used regularly, their effectiveness will be reduced as the bowel becomes used to them – and on stopping, rebound constipation can occur. Over the long term they may even trigger a non-functioning colon. Onset of action is usually rapid: within 6 to 12 hours. Stimulant laxatives should not be used by people with undiagnosed abdominal pain or vomiting in case a degree of bowel obstruction is present. They may also affect the body's salt balance. Senna is the gentlest stimulant laxative in this group. Cascara and castor oil are powerful stimulant laxatives whose use is now virtually obsolete and *not* recommended for people with IBS.

Bisacodyl
Bisacodyl tablets may cause griping abdominal pains (colic); suppositories may cause local irritation.

Tablets are usually taken at night and work within 10 to 12 hours. Suppositories are usually inserted in the morning and work within 20 to 60 minutes.

Danthron
Danthron has been linked with increased risk of liver and bowel tumours in animals. There is no evidence of a link in humans, but Danthron is only recommended for use in particular clinical situations under medical supervision (constipation in the elderly, the terminally ill or those where straining is inadvisable, such as those at risk of heart failure or heart attack). Should not be taken in pregnancy or when breastfeeding. Reported side-effects include abdominal cramps, diarrhoea, faecal incontinence, discolouration of urine and irritation of the skin around the anus after prolonged use. Act within 6 to 12 hours.

Senna
Derived from the seed pods of the plant *Senna alexandrina*, senna is a powerful laxative that usually acts within 8 to 12 hours. Usually taken at night starting with a low dose. Reserve for occasional use only – not recommended for long-term use. May trigger bowel cramps and make the symptoms of IBS worse.

Sodium Picosulphate

This powerful purgative is used to clear the bowel before an investigation such as a barium enema. It is not used to treat constipation as such. You will usually be advised to follow a low-residue (low-fibre) diet for two days before the examination and to drink copious amounts of fluid while the purgative works. Only used under medical supervision.

Phenolphthalein

A constituent of many over-the-counter preparations, phenolphthalein may cause rashes in some people and may colour alkaline urine pink.

ENEMAS

Enemas are often used when a digital rectal examination (*see page 105*) reveals impacted (hard, stuck, dehydrated) faeces in the rectum. You will be asked to lie on your left side, and the nurse or doctor may attempt to remove as much of the blockage as possible using a lubricant such as KY jelly. Most standard enemas come prepacked (100 to 150 ml fluid) in a bag or tube with a special long nozzle to assist application. Fluid will be squeezed into the back passage and you will be asked to lie in the same position for 20 to 30 minutes while the enema is absorbed to soften the motions. This is usually enough to help you push the motions out. Sometimes the bowel will not respond for several hours, especially if you have been using laxatives for years. For milder cases, a micro-enema (5 ml fluid in a tube) may be tried instead, sometimes with a couple of suppositories.

Solutions/lubricants/stimulants used in enemas include:

- arachis oil
- bisacodyl
- sodium acid phosphate
- sodium phosphate
- sodium citrate
- sodium alkylsulphoacetate

- sodium lauryl sulphoacetate
- docusate sodium
- glycerol
- sorbic acid
- sorbitol.

ANTI-DIARRHOEALS

Drugs to stop diarrhoea are mainly synthetic opiates, some of which (such as codeine) are metabolized to morphine in the body. These drugs interact with opiate receptors in the bowel to regulate smooth muscle tone and slow bowel transit time. They are useful for treating IBS symptoms in some people, especially those with functional diarrhoea. The diarrhoea associated with IBS is often worse in the early hours of the morning, between 5 and 10 a.m. ('morning rush syndrome'). In this case, an anti-diarrhoeal agent often helps if taken last thing at night and after the first bowel action every morning. Treatment should only be used for short periods of time, unless under medical supervision. Drink plenty of fluids to counter dehydration, especially if urine production has slowed down and you are only passing small amounts of dark urine.

Bulking agents (*see above*) are also ideal for use in treating diarrhoea, as they will absorb excess fluid in the gut and help to normalize bowel motions, although they may take a few days to work. Anti-diarrhoeal agents should not be used when intestinal obstruction (with overflow diarrhoea) is a possibility. If diarrhoea lasts more than a few days, check with your doctor before continuing using an anti-diarrhoeal treatment.

Codeine phosphate

Codeine phosphate acts as both an anti-diarrhoeal agent and a moderately strong painkiller. It is useful in IBS when diarrhoea is accompanied by colicky pain – but only if the diagnosis of IBS has been medically confirmed – and is therefore best used under medical supervision only. May cause nausea, vomiting, constipation, dry mouth, blurred vision or drowsiness. Should only be used occasionally, as with long-term use, tolerance and even dependence may result.

Loperamide

Loperamide is a synthetic opiate but is poorly absorbed and does not affect the central nervous system to cause drowsiness. It is the most popular drug for helping to treat diarrhoea and urgency in IBS. Possible side-effects include abdominal cramps, skin rashes, impaired bowel function (paralytic ileus) and bloating. If pregnant or breastfeeding, take only under medical supervision.

Co-phenotrope

A mixture of diphenoxylate hydrochloride (related to pethidine) and atropine sulphate. It works by slowing bowel motility and reducing fluid secretion into the gut. Usually taken every six hours until symptoms subside. Possible side-effects include allergic reactions, dry mouth, blurred vision, dizziness, nausea.

ANTI-SPASMODICS, RELAXANTS AND MOTILITY AGENTS

These drugs act directly on the smooth muscle of the gut to prevent spasm. They are not successful for everyone and can produce undesirable side-effects. They should not be taken for undiagnosed abdominal pain or bloating in case a degree of intestinal obstruction is present. Should not be taken during pregnancy or when breastfeeding except under medical supervision.

Alverine Citrate

An anti-spasmodic agent useful for treating smooth muscle spasm in IBS, and painful periods. Possible side-effects include nausea, headache, itching, skin rashes or dizziness.

Cisapride

Cisapride is thought to work by increasing the release of a natural nerve chemical (acetylcholine) within the network of nerves supplying the gut wall. It is classed as a motility (prokinetic) agent as it co-ordinates bowel contractions so they become functional rather than capable only of squashing bowel contents ineffectually. It is prescribed to treat delayed gastric emptying and also to prevent acid reflux from the stomach up into the gullet (heartburn or reflux oesophagitis). Cisapride has been shown to increase bowel frequency in some people with constipation, and is currently under investigation as a possible treatment for irritable bowel syndrome.

Possible side-effects include abdominal cramps, increased bowel noises, diarrhoea, headache, light-headedness and urinary frequency. Very rarely, fits have been reported.

Dicyclomine

Dicyclomine is taken three times a day before or after meals. It has a direct action on the smooth muscle lining the gut to stop excessive contraction. This relieves spasm without affecting normal gastric motility. It relieves colicky abdominal pain, cramps, persistent non-specific diarrhoea (with or without altering constipation) and flatulence. Should not be taken (except under medical supervision) by those with glaucoma, an enlarged prostate gland, or a hiatus hernia associated with reflux oesophagitis (indigestion) as it may make symptoms worse. Possible side-effects include dry mouth, thirst, dizziness, blurred vision, tiredness, drowsiness, rash, constipation, anorexia, nausea, headache or painful urination (dysuria).

Mebeverine

Mebeverine is taken three times a day, 20 minutes before meals. It works in precisely the same way as dicyclomine. After a period of several weeks, when symptoms have improved, the dose can be slowly reduced. No significant side-effects have been reported.

Propantheline

This anti-spasmodic agent is useful for treating smooth muscle spasm and abdominal pain in IBS, and for urinary frequency. Usually taken three times per day before meals and at bedtime. Should not be taken by people with glaucoma or an enlarged prostate gland. Should only be used under medical supervision in people with heart, nerve, liver or kidney disease. Possible side-effects include dry mouth, blurred vision, dizziness, flushing, difficulty passing water or constipation. Rarely, skin rashes, fever or mental confusion have been reported.

Peppermint Oil

Peppermint oil has a direct relaxant effect on intestinal smooth muscle and helps to relieve pain, bloating, distension and wind. Capsules are taken 30 minutes before meals and may be used for up to three months. Do not break or chew the capsules, as it is important that the oil passes down to the large bowel to produce its medicinal effect. May cause heartburn or a burning sensation around the anus, in which case cut back on the dose.

ANTIDEPRESSANTS

For patients who are resistant to other types of treatment, a type of drug called a tricyclic antidepressant often produces good results. Although you are being treated with an antidepressant, this does not necessarily mean your doctor thinks you are depressed. The way in which these drugs work in IBS is not fully understood. It may be that they increase the quantity of neurotransmitters (nerve communication chemicals) in nerve endings in the gut to reduce gut mobility and spasm, or to decrease pain perception. If your doctor prescribes an antidepressant tablet for you, ask how long you will need to take it and what the possible side-effects are.

SURGERY

It was recently found that IBS sufferers who had had a surgical operation to remove co-incidental haemorrhoids noticed a significant improvement in their IBS symptoms – the success rate was almost 100 per cent. It is thought that the procedure involved interrupted the normal anal reflexes that can trigger spasm in the rest of the gut. In certain conditions, the mucous lining of the rectum above the anus may droop (prolapse) and irritate the anal margin. This irritation is interpreted as a bowel motion waiting to be voided, and a reflex signal triggers contractions to expel it. This in turn pushes the loose mucous lining further into the anus and triggers even more contraction and spasm. By removing the loose rectal lining during the haemorrhoid operation, this vicious circle unwinds and the bowel returns to normal motility. The operation may also involve cutting small nerves to prevent feedback hyperstimulation of the gut. At present, the operation is only available for treating haemorrhoids, but is being evaluated further with a view to helping people with IBS. The operation has three stages:

1 Up to 15 elastic (Baron's) bands are applied to take up the slack in the loose, prolapsing mucous lining of the rectum
2 The internal anal sphincter is cut slightly to loosen it and prevent spasm (lateral sphincterotomy) – it may also be gently stretched and dilated to paralyse the muscle partially and to reduce its contractile strength during healing
3 External anal skin tags and varicose veins (piles, haemorrhoids) are removed using small radial cuts.

Surgical removal of haemorrhoids is quite painful unfortunately and you will usually need to stay in hospital until you can open your bowels with the help of laxatives. Painkillers and warm baths will help to ease discomfort, but complete healing takes three to six weeks.

Chapter Nine

COMPLEMENTARY THERAPIES

Many sufferers from irritable bowel syndrome seek help from alternative therapies. There can be many reasons for this. Once a diagnosis of IBS is made, some sufferers are left feeling that their doctor has lost interest in their symptoms as nothing more serious has been found, or that their problems are due to an emotional cause – in either case, the holistic approach followed by alternative practitioners can help. In addition, orthodox medicine can offer little in the way of permanent relief of symptoms, and some patients find very little temporary relief from their doctor's prescriptions. IBS is a long-term (chronic) problem with symptoms that may come and go over a long period of time, leaving the sufferer constantly searching for new remedies to try: alternative treatments are often helpful in relieving these symptoms.

Before trying alternative treatments for your symptoms, make sure you have been fully investigated and the diagnosis of IBS confirmed by your doctor. Several different bowel diseases can produce similar symptoms, so it is important to seek medical advice for any new problem that continues for more than a week or so. Irritable bowel syndrome is not a diagnosis you should make or attempt to treat yourself, as you may risk overlooking a more serious condition.

When choosing an alternative practitioner, bear in mind that standards of training and experience vary widely. Where possible:

■ Select a therapist on the basis of personal recommendation from a satisfied client whom you know and whose opinion you trust.

- Check what qualifications the therapist has, and check his or her standing with the relevant umbrella organization for that therapy. The organization will be able to tell you what training their members have undertaken and their code of ethics, and can refer you to qualified practitioners in your area.
- Find out how long your course of treatment will last and how much it is likely to cost.
- Ask how much experience the therapist has had in treating IBS, and what his or her rate of success is.

The following complementary therapies have helped many people with IBS but, just as with orthodox medicine, not every treatment will suit every individual.

ACUPUNCTURE

Acupuncture is based on the belief that life energy (*Chi* or *Qi*) flows through the body along 12 different channels called meridians. When this energy flow becomes blocked, symptoms of illness are triggered. By inserting fine needles into specific acupuncture points overlying these meridians, blockages are overcome and the flow of Chi corrected or altered to relieve symptoms. Altogether, there are 365 acupoints in the body; your therapist will select which points to use depending on your individual symptoms. Fine, disposable needles are used, which cause little if any discomfort. You may notice a slight pricking sensation, or an odd tingling buzz as the needle is inserted a few millimetres into the skin. The needles are usually left in place for up to 20 minutes, and may be twiddled periodically. Sometimes a small cone of dried herbs is ignited and burned near the active acupoint to warm the skin. This is known as moxibustion. The best known effect of Chi manipulation is in pain relief (local anaesthesia). Research suggests that acupuncture causes the release of natural, heroin-like chemicals in the body which act as natural painkillers. Acupuncture can be effective in treating many of the symptoms of irritable bowel syndrome, including constipation, diarrhoea and cramping pains.

Acupressure is similar to acupuncture, but instead of inserting needles at selected points along the meridians, firm thumb pressure or fingertip massage is used to stimulate them. The best known example of acupressure is Shiatsu massage.

AROMATHERAPY MASSAGE

Abdominal massage is often beneficial in getting a constipated bowel moving, relieving wind and distension, or easing the pain associated with diarrhoea. You can do this yourself or visit a qualified aromatherapist. Before a massage, you may find it helpful to apply alternating hot and cold compresses to your abdomen, to stimulate the local circulation. Some therapists also recommend that you drink a glass of hot water containing a few drops of the essential oils ginger and fennel, sweetened with honey, 20 minutes before you have a massage.

If you choose to try giving yourself an abdominal massage, use firm circular movements. A diluted aromatherapy oil can be used in a dilution of 10–20 drops essential oil to 30 ml (1 tablespoon) carrier oil (such as almond or grapeseed). As a general aromatherapy massage for someone with irritable bowel syndrome, the best oils to use are rosemary and marjoram, singly or together, to which a little oil of black pepper or fennel can be added. Oils can also be selected for use singly or in combination depending on your main symptoms (*NB:* Substitute rose oil for rosemary oil if you have high blood pressure, and avoid fennel oil if you suffer from epilepsy):

FOR CONSTIPATION

- black pepper (use sparingly)
- cardamom
- cedarwood (not to be used during pregnancy)
- fennel (do not use if you suffer from epilepsy)
- ginger
- lemon
- patchouli
- peppermint (not to be used during pregnancy)

- rosemary (do not use if you suffer from high blood pressure or epilepsy)
- sandalwood

FOR WIND AND DISTENSION

- cardamom
- coriander
- dill
- peppermint (not to be used during pregnancy)
- spearmint

FOR DIARRHOEA

- basil
- camomile
- lavender (not to be used during first three months of pregnancy)
- lemon
- marjoram (not to be used during pregnancy)
- orange
- peppermint (not to be used during pregnancy)

FOR COLICKY, LOWER ABDOMINAL PAIN

- camomile (not to be used during first three months of pregnancy)
- clove
- cypress (not to be used during pregnancy)
- eucalyptus
- ginger
- lavender (not to be used during first three months of pregnancy)
- neroli
- patchouli
- peppermint (not to be used during pregnancy)
- rosemary (do not use if you suffer from epilepsy or high blood pressure)
- thyme (not to be used during pregnancy)

Place the container of diluted oil in a bowl of warm water to heat it gently, so it is comfortable to use on your skin.

Make sure it has been at least an hour or so since your last meal. Lie down in a warm, quiet room with the curtains pulled. Expose your abdomen, but make sure you have a towel, blanket, or duvet over your legs and chest to keep you warm.

Place some warmed oil on your hands and gently massage around your abdomen. Move in a clockwise direction, starting on the lower right-hand side by the groin, just above your pubic hair. Massage with slow, circular movements of your hand, pressing as deeply as you can without causing discomfort. Work your way up to the lower rib cage, across your upper abdomen and down the left-hand side to your groin again. All together, the massage should last around 15 minutes. It may be easier (and more pleasant and relaxing!) for a partner, relative or friend to do this for you.

COLONIC IRRIGATION

This procedure aims to remove impacted waste matter from the folds in the colonic wall, in the hope that by removing harmful bowel bacteria, beneficial species such as *Lactobacillus acidophilus* will proliferate better. Although the technique is excellent for overcoming constipation, it may trigger IBS symptoms in some sufferers by stretching the large bowel and encouraging reflex spasm.

During the procedure, which is similar to an enema, the practitioner will insert a lubricated tube into your rectum. Water is pumped into the lower bowel and a special valve drains waste fluid away down a separate part of the tube. The process takes around half an hour and may leave you feeling light-headed afterwards.

ELECTRODE THERAPY

Electrodes can be attached to the anus to cure severe constipation. They help sufferers learn to co-ordinate and relax their pelvic floor muscles by showing how muscle contraction and relaxation affect the tone of the bowel. Between three and six weekly sessions lasting one hour each are usually needed.

HERBALISM

Many edible natural herbs and spices commonly found in the kitchen can calm the gut, relieve painful spasms and help to prevent wind distension and bloating. These include:

- angelica
- aniseed
- black pepper
- caraway
- camomile
- clove
- dill
- fennel
- ginger
- lemon balm
- marjoram
- parsley
- peppermint
- rosemary
- spearmint.

Use them as a garnish on food or as soothing, herbal teas. Plain infusions of camomile or peppermint are available in teabags, as are delicious combinations such as camomile and spearmint or fennel and lemon balm.

Ginger

Ginger helps to reduce flatulence and nausea, and relaxes the smooth muscle lining the gut to relieve spasm. Can be taken in a dose of 500–1000 mg as a powder, or as 2 drops concentrated extract three times per day.

Peppermint

Peppermint essential oil is rich in menthol, which relaxes excessive spasm of the smooth muscle lining the digestive tract. To relieve mild intestinal cramps or flatulence, drink peppermint tea. Where symptoms are more severe, peppermint gives the most benefit if it can reach the colon undigested, and is therefore best taken in the form of enteric-coated capsules. These prevent the release of the peppermint oil until it has reached the large bowel. Treatment may produce a warm, tingling feeling in the back passage due to some of the essential oil not being absorbed. This is not harmful and will usually disappear if you cut back on the dosage you are taking.

Garlic

Garlic is often used to treat diarrhoea, wind and indigestion, although if raw cloves are eaten excessively, they can actually produce flatulence. Enteric-coated tablets or powder extracts can be taken at a dose of around 900 mg per day and may improve symptoms. Garlic also has the additional benefits of lowering high blood pressure, changing blood fat ratios to reduce the risk of heart disease, and improving blood flow to the extremities and brain.

Medical Herbalism

Many non-culinary herbs, including those used by Chinese practitioners, have medicinal effects. Most are available as tablets, capsules, dried extracts, concentrated drops and tinctures (concentrated liquid extracts, often preserved in alcohol) from chemists, healthfood shops or herbal practitioners.

For painful bowel spasm, herbs with a natural anti-spasmodic effect include:

- camomile
- dioscera
- hops
- lobelia
- lemon balm (Melissa)
- marsh-mallow
- meadowsweet
- mistletoe
- pasque flowers
- skull cap
- valerian
- viburnum
- wild yam.

To make your own spasm-relieving tincture, try mixing 30g of meadowsweet with 30g of marsh-mallow root, 15g of hops and 15g of camomile flowers. Add 1.5 litres of boiling water, cover and simmer for 15 minutes. Allow to cool, then strain. Take 3–4 tablespoons before each meal.

For constipation, herbs with a natural laxative effect include:

- aloe (can have a powerful effect)
- balmony
- baldo
- barberry
- buckthorn (powerful: use sparingly)
- cascara sagrada (powerful: use sparingly)
- cassia
- chinese angelica
- dandelion root (also has a diuretic effect)
- fennel
- ginger
- goldenseal
- linseed (bulking and lubricating)
- liquorice (do not take if you suffer from fluid retention or high blood pressure)

- marsh-mallow root
- psyllium husks (bulking laxative)
- rhubarb root (powerful: use sparingly)
- senna leaves (powerful: use sparingly)
- wahoo
- yellow dock.

For constipation that is an ongoing (chronic) problem, gentler herbs such as ginger or dandelion root are better than stronger ones such as buckthorn. Goldenseal helps to normalize muscular action in the bowel, and is therefore advised by some practitioners to treat either constipation or diarrhoea in IBS.

For diarrhoea, herbs with a natural anti-diarrhoeal effect include:

- slippery elm
- goldenseal
- barberry
- poria.

The latter two are mainly useful against infective diarrhoea rather than the functional diarrhoea that occurs with IBS. Some sufferers find them helpful, however. Goldenseal helps to normalize muscular action in the bowel, and is therefore advised by some practitioners to treat diarrhoea as well as constipation in IBS.

For bloating, herbs that can ease gaseous distension and help bowel movement include:

- angelic root
- aniseed
- calamus
- caraway
- cardamom
- cayenne
- camomile
- coriander
- dandelion root
- fennel

- ginger
- magnolia bark
- peppermint
- thyme.

Doses of the above herbs vary. Check packaging for details of how much to use per day.

Aloe Vera

Many sufferers swear by Aloe vera for relieving symptoms of IBS. The plant looks similar to a cactus but actually belongs to the lily family. There are many species, of which *Aloe barbadensis* is reputed to have the most useful medicinal properties.

Aloe gel is squeezed from the succulent leaves, which can grow to over 60 cm long. This contains a unique mix of vitamins, amino acids, enzymes and minerals that have been valued for their healing properties for over 6,000 years. When diluted to form a juice, the extract is said to increase energy and is widely used to help a wide range of illnesses, including irritable bowel syndrome and problems such as oral thrush, heartburn, gastritis (inflammation of the stomach), peptic ulcers, constipation, Crohn's disease, colitis (inflammation of the colon), diverticulitis, haemorrhoids (piles) and threadworms. It is also used to help treat several skin conditions, arthritis, and ME.

Aloe vera gel contains soapy substances (saponins) that help to cleanse the bowel, and pulpy microfibres (lignins) whose fibre content helps to absorb fluid and toxins from the bowel and bulk up the motions. It contains substances that:

- are anti-inflammatory (anthraquinones and natural plant steroids)
- hasten wound healing (fibroblast growth factor)
- are powerful antioxidants (vitamins C, E, betacarotene)
- are antiseptic (saponins and anthraquinones), helping to kill some bacteria, viruses and fungi.

Aloe vera juice can be made from fresh liquid extract (gel) or from powdered aloe. The fresh gel has to be stabilized within hours of harvesting to prevent oxidation and de-activation. When selecting a product, aim for one made from 100 per cent pure aloe vera. Its strength needs to be at least 40 per cent by volume to be effective (ideally approaching 95 per cent). Also, choose one that is made from Aloe liquid rather than powder. You may find it more palatable to choose a product containing a little natural fruit juice (such as grape, apple) to improve the flavour, although some sufferers find that fruit juice makes their symptoms worse. Sufferers have found relief from symptoms by taking as little as 15–50 ml aloe gel/juice per day. Start off with a small dose (such as 1 teaspoon) and work up to around 1–2 tablespoons per day to find the dose that suits you best. Aloe has a powerful cathartic effect; taking too much will produce a brisk laxative response.

Some women using Aloe vera notice that it increases their menstrual flow. Aloe vera stimulates uterine contractions, and for this reason should not be used during pregnancy. Similarly, it should be avoided when breastfeeding as its active ingredients are excreted in breastmilk and can produce diarrhoea in the infant.

Evening Primrose Oil

The beautiful evening primrose flower only blooms for a single day, but a valuable oil can be extracted from its seeds to provide one of the most popular and useful food supplements available. It can help a wide range of problems from dry itchy skin, eczema, psoriasis and acne to pre-menstrual syndrome, menopausal problems and cyclical breast pain. It has also proved useful in the treatment of irritable bowel syndrome, rheumatoid arthritis, high cholesterol levels and high blood pressure.

Evening primrose oil is a rich source of an essential fatty acid (EFA) called GLA (gamma linolenic acid – sometimes shortened to gamolenic acid). The body can synthesize some GLA from other essential fatty acids in the diet, but as many people do not obtain enough of these important substances, it is common to be deficient in GLA.

There are three essential fatty acids:

1 linolenic acid (of which one type is gamma-linolenic acid)
2 linoleic acid
3 arachidonic acid (can be synthesized from linolenic or linoleic acids)

DIETARY SOURCES OF ESSENTIAL FATTY ACIDS

- Linoleic acid alone is found in sunflower seed, almonds, corn, sesame seed, safflower oil and extra virgin olive oil.
- Linolenic acid alone is found in evening primrose oil, starflower (borage) seed oil and blackcurrant seed oil.
- Both linoleic and linolenic acids are found in rich quantities in walnuts, pumpkin seeds, soybeans, linseed oil, rapeseed oil and flax oil.
- Arachidonic acid is found in many foods (such as seafood, meat, dairy products) and can also be made from linoleic or linolenic acids.

Dietary essential fatty acids, including GLA, are metabolized in the body to form hormone-like substances known as prostaglandins. Prostaglandins are found in all body tissues and play a major role in regulating inflammation, blood clotting and hormone balance; they are also involved in the immune responses involved in infections, chronic inflammatory diseases and even cancer.

THE EFA PATHWAY

Linoleic acid → Gamma-linolenic acid (GLA) (evening primrose oil) → dihomo-gamma linolenic acid → arachidonic acid → prostaglandins

---

If your diet is lacking in GLA, it can be synthesized from dietary linoleic acid, but this reaction relies on a particular enzyme (delta-6-desaturase) which is easily blocked by a number of factors, including:

- eating too much saturated (animal) fat
- eating too many trans-fatty acids (such as found in margarines)

- eating too much sugar
- drinking too much alcohol
- deficiency of vitamins and minerals, especially vitamin B_6, zinc and magnesium
- increasing age
- crash dieting
- smoking cigarettes
- exposure to pollution.

When you do not get enough essential fatty acids from your diet, the metabolism can make do with the next best fatty acids available (such as those derived from saturated animal fats), but as a result prostaglandin imbalances are common. This is because prostaglandins made from other sorts of fat cannot be converted into the same type of prostaglandins made from the three essential fatty acids. This imbalance is thought to increase the risk of developing inflammatory diseases, hormonal imbalances, blood clots and dry, itchy skin. It has also been implicated in IBS where there seems to be a relative increase in inflammatory PGE2 prostaglandins and lack of PGE1 prostaglandins, especially in patients suffering from diarrhoea.

Taking an evening primrose oil supplement provides dietary GLA and feeds into the EFA pathway, bypassing any enzyme blocks and helping to correct any prostaglandin or hormone imbalances.

When choosing an evening primrose oil (EPO) supplement:

- Select one containing 100 per cent pure EPO.
- Choose one containing at least 500 mg EPO per capsule plus some vitamin E, which helps to protect the GLA content from oxidation and boosts its function.
- Certain vitamins and minerals are needed during the metabolism of essential fatty acids. These are vitamin C, vitamin B_6, vitamin B_3 (niacin), zinc and magnesium. If you are taking evening primrose oil, make sure your intake of these vitamins and minerals is adequate.

For general preventive health, take 500–1000 mg EPO per day. For treating a specific condition, you need to take 3000–4000 mg per day for at least three months before you will be able to tell if it is producing a beneficial effect. Some evidence suggests that EPO supplement are best taken in the late afternoon, between 4 and 6 p.m.

Taking too much EPO may cause mild diarrhoea. Some women taking high-dose supplements may notice breast enlargement or a change in their normal period pattern. If you suffer from temporal lobe epilepsy (an uncommon nervous disorder), only take EPO under medical supervision.

Ginseng

Siberian ginseng (*Eleutherococcus senticosus*) is used extensively to improve stamina and strength, particularly during or after illness. It seems to help the body adapt when under physical or emotional stress, and boosts immunity. When given to 13,000 workers at a Russian car factory, the number of days off work due to health problems dropped by a third. Siberian ginseng – and related roots such as Korean ginseng (*Panax ginseng*) and American ginseng (*Ginseng quinquefolium*) – are useful herbal supplements to take when you are feeling under the weather, or suffering from a relapse of symptoms that are dragging you down.

Dose: 0.2–1g three times a day

HOMOEOPATHY

Homoeopathic medicine is based on the belief that natural substances can boost the body's own healing powers to relieve the symptoms and signs of illness. Natural substances are selected which, if used full-strength, would produce symptoms in a healthy person similar to those it is designed to treat. This is the first principle of homoeopathy, that 'Like cures Like.'

The second major principle of homoeopathy is that increasing the dilution of a solution has the opposite effect, that is, increases its potency ('Less Cures More'). By diluting noxious and even poisonous substances many millions of times, their healing properties are enhanced while their undesirable side-effects are lost.

On the centesimal scale, dilutions of 100^{-6} (1 drop tincture mixed with 99 drops of alcohol or water and shaken; this is then done a further six times, each time 1 drop of the dilution being added to 99 drops of alcohol or water) are described as potencies of 6c, dilutions of 100^{-30} are written as a potency of 30c, etc. To illustrate just how diluted these substances are, a dilution of 12c (100^{-12}) is comparable to a pinch of salt dissolved in the same amount of water as is found in the Atlantic Ocean!

Homoeopathy is thought to work in a dynamic way, boosting your body's own healing powers. The principles 'like cures like' and 'less cures more' are difficult concepts to accept, yet convincing trials have shown that homoeopathy is significantly better than placebos in treating many chronic (long-term) conditions including hayfever, asthma and rheumatoid arthritis.

Homoeopathic remedies should ideally be taken on their own, at least 30 minutes either before or after eating or drinking. Tablets should also be taken without handling them first – tip them into the lid of the container, or onto a teaspoon to transfer them into your mouth. Then suck or chew them, don't swallow them whole.

Homoeopathic treatments are prescribed according to your symptoms rather than any particular disease, so two patients with the same label of 'irritable bowel syndrome' who have different symptoms will need different homoeopathic treatments.

Homoeopathic remedies may be prescribed by a medically-trained homoeopathic doctor on a normal NHS prescription form and dispensed by homoeopathic pharmacists for the usual prescription charge or exemptions. Alternatively, you can consult a private homoeopathic practitioner or buy remedies direct from the pharmacist.

Although it is best to see a trained homoeopath who can assess your constitutional type, personality, lifestyle, family background, likes and dislikes as well as your symptoms before deciding which treatment is right for you, you may find the following remedies helpful. After taking the remedies for the time stated, if there is no obvious improvement consult a practitioner. Don't be surprised if your symptoms initially get worse before they get better – persevere through this common reaction to treatment – it is a good sign which shows the remedy is working.

- For constipation with little desire to open the bowels: *Alumina 6c.* (Take every 2 hours for up to 10 doses)
- For constipation with spasm and strong urges to open the bowels: *Nux vomica 6c.* (Take every 2 hours for up to 10 doses)
- For constipation with large, hard, dry, crumbling motions: *Bryonia 6c.* (Take 4 times a day for up to 5 days)
- For diarrhoea with flatulence or burning in the rectum and anus: *Aloe 6c.* (Take hourly for up to 10 doses)
- For diarrhoea with anxiety and stress: *Argentum nit. 6c.* (Take every half an hour for up to 10 doses)
- For diarrhoea with anal itching or soreness plus foul-smelling wind: *Sulphur 6c.* (Take every half an hour for up to 10 doses)
- For alternating constipation and diarrhoea, with flatulence, colicky pain and passing mucus in the stools: *Argentum nit. 6c.* (Take 4 times a day for up to 14 days)
- For colic with exhausting diarrhoea and excessive flatulence: *China 6c.* (Take every 15 minutes for up to 8 doses)
- For nausea, tearing pains and watery stools with mucus and loss of appetite: *Colchicum 6c.* (Take 4 times a day for up to 14 days)
- For profuse diarrhoea with burning or colicky abdominal pains, restlessness, anxiety and chills: *Arsenicum album 6c.* (Take every 15 minutes for up to 8 doses)
- For green-tinged diarrhoea with abdominal rumbling and stomach cramps which are worse in the morning: *Podophyllum 6c.* (Take every 15 minutes for up to 8 doses)
- For profuse, strong-smelling, burning diarrhoea and an increased sensitivity to temperature changes: *Merc. sol. 6c.* (Take every 15 minutes for up to 8 doses)
- For simple diarrhoea associated with IBS, especially if symptoms are brought on by drinking coffee: *Psorinum 6c.* (Take 4 times a day for up to 14 days)
- For gripping bowel pains, which improve when doubled up: *Colocynthis 6c or 30c.* (Take 4 times a day for up to 14 days)
- For sudden, colicky or shooting pains (especially on the right-hand side of the abdomen) which may be accompanied by bloating and are made better by doubling

up or applying warmth, and are made worse by cold: *Mag. phos. 6c.* (Take every 5 minutes for up to 10 doses)

- For bloating and distension, especially after eating or when constipated: *Lycopodium 6c.* (Take every half an hour for up to 10 doses)
- For back pain and a sense of spasm and coldness round the umbilical region, with or without nausea or diarrhoea: *Terebinth 6c.* (Take 4 times a day for up to 14 days)
- For IBS symptoms, especially violent vomiting and diarrhoea, associated with cramps in the calves, headaches and menstrual problems or during pregnancy: *Verat. alb. 6c.* (Take every 4 hours for up to 7 days)

Bach Rescue Remedy

Bach Rescue Remedy is a homoeopathic preparation designed to help you cope with life's ups and downs, and to reduce the physical and emotional symptoms of stress and chronic illness such as irritable bowel syndrome. It contains five flower essences: Cherry Plum, Clematis, Impatiens, Rock Rose, and Star of Bethlehem, preserved in brandy. Add 4 drops of Rescue Remedy to a glass of water and sip slowly, every three to five minutes, holding the liquid in your mouth for a while before swallowing. Alternatively, place 4 drops directly under your tongue. Useful for acute recurrences of symptoms that leave you feeling unable to cope.

After completing a course of homoeopathy, you will usually feel much better in yourself with a greatly improved sense of well-being that lets you cope with any remaining symptoms in a much more positive way.

HYPNOTHERAPY

Hypnotherapy can be effective in relieving the symptoms of IBS. Research shows that it can significantly reduce abdominal pain and distension, encourage a regular bowel and improve general well-being after just a short course of treatment.

A gastroenterologist and hypnotherapist together studied 32 patients with severe, refractory IBS. After eight weekly hypnotherapy sessions lasting 30 minutes each, the sufferers achieved a stable improvement in symptoms.

The hypnotherapist asked sufferers to place their hands on their abdomens and induce feelings of warmth and comfort in this area. He then made several suggestions related to symptom reduction and control over gut function. This was reinforced with visual imagery, and self-hypnosis tapes were provided for daily use. Overall, patients found that their abdominal pain and distension went from being moderately severe to only mild or even non-existent.

NATUROPATHY

Many patients have found that live yoghurt eaten every day relieves their symptoms. The Lactobacilli bacteria in live (Bio) yoghurt can happily line your bowel and keep it healthy and regular – they seem to survive the passage through stomach acids in enough numbers to recolonize the bowel. Eat at least one carton (150 ml) of low-fat live yoghurt containing *Lactobacillus acidophilus* per day. In addition, you may also benefit from a yoghurt-like liquid supplement containing *Lactobacillus casei* Shirota. This (sold as Yakult) was developed by a team of scientists in Europe to replenish the bowel with a healthy, human strain of *Lactobacillus*.

Other Dietary Tips

Follow a wholefood diet containing more brown bread, brown rice, cereals, salads, fresh fruit and vegetables for roughage – take apples, bananas, pears, grapes, dried apricots or figs into work for snacking on rather than crisps or biscuits. Soak five or six prunes in water or cold tea overnight and eat for breakfast with natural yoghurt.

Molasses is an effective and harmless laxative – take 1–2 teaspoons daily.

REFLEXOLOGY

This technique was used in China over 5,000 years ago and was also popular with the ancient Egyptians. Reflexology is based on the principle that points in the feet – known as reflexes – are indirectly related to other parts of the body. Massage over these reflexes can detect areas of tenderness and subtle textural changes which help to pinpoint problems in various organs, including the gut. By working on these tender spots with tiny pressure movements, nerves are thought to be stimulated that pass messages to distant organs and relieve symptoms. Some people with IBS have found reflexology helpful.

SILICIC ACID

Silicon is one of the commonest elements on Earth, coming second only to oxygen. It makes up 40 per cent of the Earth's crust and is found in a variety of substances including brick, cement, glass, quartz, emeralds, silicon chips and even non-stick frying pans. The foods with the richest content of silicon include wholegrain wheat, potatoes and unprocessed barley, oats and rye.

Although silicon in its pure form is biologically inactive, it is now recognized as an essential trace element. In its soluble (colloidal) state, silicic acid, it is essential for normal growth and development. Silicic acid occurs naturally in low concentrations in most food and water. More and more people are now using colloidal silicic acid as a health supplement.

Colloidal silicic acid can be helpful in treating the symptoms of IBS. It comes in the form of a gel which, when taken internally, reduces symptoms of bloating, flatulence and irregular bowel habit, especially diarrhoea. It has also proved helpful for more serious bowel problems, such as ulcerative colitis and Crohn's Disease.

As well as protecting the intestinal tract, silicic acid can soothe mouth ulcers and inflamed gums (gingivitis). It lines the stomach, absorbs toxins and irritants, and protects an inflamed stomach lining from self-digestion with stomach acid. It is therefore effective in the treatment of acid indigestion (gastritis) and heartburn due to acid reflux up into the gullet (reflux oesophagitis). It is safe to use during pregnancy.

Silicic acid should be taken in a dose of 1 tablespoon daily (30 ml) per day, diluted with fruit juice if preferred.

VISUALIZATION

When you feel an attack of pain coming on, try visualization to aid relaxation and relieve your distress. Stop what you are doing and sit down somewhere private and quiet. Close your eyes and, instead of focusing on your pain, imagine yourself:

- walking through a sunlit forest glade, with the sound of gently running water and bird song surrounding you, while a cool breeze ruffles your hair
- swimming in a warm tropical ocean next to a white-sand, deserted beach
- sitting in the sun on the veranda of a log chalet high up on a snow-crested mountain – breathe in the cool air and hear the soft drip of snow melting from the surrounding fir trees.

Visualization has been shown to help bowel problems including inflammatory bowel disease and irritable bowel syndrome, as well as aiding relaxation.

Chapter Ten

DIET AND LIFESTYLE TIPS

Even if you don't want to follow a strict eating regime, there are several simple diet and lifestyle changes that will help to improve your IBS symptoms.

EXERCISE

Regular exercise, especially in the open air, is beneficial in helping IBS symptoms. As well as burning off stress hormones, it stimulates production of the body's own natural painkillers, endorphins and enkephalins. Exercise, therefore, seems to help reduce the discomfort of IBS and improve overall mood. Exercise also hastens bowel emptying and can relieve bloating and distension. Aim to exercise for at least half an hour, three times per week – enough to raise a 'glow', get your pulse pounding and leave you feeling slightly breathless.

DIET AND LIFESTYLE

- Follow the old advice: Breakfast like a king, lunch like a lord and dine like a pauper.
- Eat meals in an unrushed fashion – leave plenty of time to eat so you don't bolt down your food and swallow excessive amounts of air.
- Sit down to eat rather than grabbing a snack on the hoof.
- Try eating several small meals spread throughout the day rather than the traditional three large meals with little in between.

- Cut out all pre-packaged or processed foods and stick to a natural, whole-food diet.
- Eat more complex, unrefined carbohydrates which contain a variety of fibre types such as wholegrain bread, wholemeal pasta, brown rice and unsweetened wholegrain breakfast cereals such as muesli or porridge.
- Eat more fresh fruit and vegetables – especially nuts, seeds, figs, apricots, prunes, peas, sweetcorn and beans.
- If bran seems to make your symptoms worse – even after persevering with it for two or three weeks – concentrate on getting fibre from vegetables, rice and fruit. Try supplements containing ispaghula, psyllium or sterculia, but alternate these – don't use just one all the time or you will lose the benefits (*see page 76*).
- Cut down on the amount of saturated fat in your diet. Avoid dairy products such as butter, cream and whole-fat milk. Instead, try semi-skimmed or skimmed milk and olive-oil based products in place of butter. Low-fat fromage frais is a delicious and healthy substitute for cream.
- Try adding live yoghurt (containing a culture of *Lactobacillus acidophilus*) or a drink containing *Lactobacillus casei* Shirota (Yakult) to your diet. Lactobacilli have been shown to survive stomach acids and can colonize the bowel – in some people, they can damp down IBS symptoms.
- Cut back on your intake of red meat to see if this improves your symptoms. Eat more fish and skinless white meat instead.
- Don't fry or roast your food – grill, bake, casserole or steam it instead.
- Many natural herbs and spices contain substances that calm the bowels, relieve spasm and prevent a build-up of wind. These include aniseed, camomile, lemon balm, clove, dill, fennel, black pepper, marjoram, parsley, peppermint, rosemary and spearmint. Use them as a garnish on food or as soothing, herbal teas. (*For more on herbs, see Chapter 9.*)
- If wind is a problem, avoid beans, cabbage and any other foods which encourage bacterial fermentation and may trigger intestinal gas.
- Avoid sugar, cakes, sweets and chocolate.

- Some people find that spicy food irritates their bowel lining and makes symptoms worse. Try eating lots of spicy foods one week, then cutting them out the next to see if your symptoms change.
- Some people with IBS are sensitive to acid foods such as oranges, grapefruit, tomatoes and vinegar. Again, try cutting them out to see if this helps.
- Try to avoid caffeine-containing drinks such as tea, coffee and some soft drinks. Some people are also sensitive to resins in coffee beans, so you may find that drinking decaffeinated coffee can still upset you.
- Try to avoid drinking alcohol, which has a direct irritant effect on the gut.
- Avoid artificial sweeteners such as sorbitol, which are not easily digested and can make symptoms of IBS worse.
- Stop smoking, and try to avoid passive smoking too. There are receptors in the gut which react with nicotine and cause the bowel to constrict, making symptoms worse.
- Try to avoid unnecessary stress. The bowel contains receptors that interact with stress hormones, which will make spasm and diarrhoea worse. For example, if driving in heavy traffic winds you up, avoid this as much as you can. Leave plenty of time for journeys, do more walking or try to avoid rush-hours.
- Visit the toilet regularly throughout the day, whenever the urge strikes. Don't put voiding off because you are too busy. Try to retrain your bowels into a regular habit.
- Don't strain to empty your bowels. If necessary, use a little petroleum jelly or water-based gel as a lubricant.
- Drink more fluids – especially bottled water or herbal teas. Aim to drink 2–3 litres of fluid per day.

Dietary Changes to Help Diarrhoea

- Avoid eating too much raw or dried fruit.
- Avoid spicy foods.
- Cut back on caffeine intake.
- Avoid artificial sweeteners (especially sorbitol and mannitol).

- Drink plenty of fluids (especially water) to prevent dehydration.
- Eating a live (BIO) yoghurt containing *Lactobacillus acidophilus* can help to replenish the normal bacterial flora of the bowel.
- Eating bananas seems to help.

Dietary Changes to Help Constipation

- In general, aim to eat more fresh fruit, vegetables, salads and pulses.
- Fibre-rich pulses include peas, beans, lentils and chick-peas.
- Eat more fibre-rich dried fruits – especially figs – and seeds – especially sunflower, pumpkin, fenugreek, fennel and linseed. Buy in small quantities with a reasonable sell-by date. Add to salads and yoghurt for an extra crunch.
- Eat more wholegrain cereals: oats, brown rice, wholewheat pasta, wholegrain bread, whole rye, buckwheat, millet, bulgar wheat and couscous.
- Aim to drink one glass (350 ml) water before each meal, plus another two or three between meals to bulk up your fibre-rich diet.
- Consider taking a vitamin and mineral supplement containing calcium, magnesium, vitamin C and the B-complex vitamins.
- Natural laxatives include figs, prunes, pears, rhubarb, molasses and linseed.

A Stricter Eating Regime

Try eliminating dairy products from your diet for a week to see if this helps – some people diagnosed as having IBS may have lactose intolerance instead (*see page 83*). While avoiding dairy products or restricting your diet in any way, take a good vitamin and mineral supplement containing calcium. If your symptoms do improve, ask your doctor whether you need investigations for lactose intolerance. Also request dietary advice from a nutritionist to ensure you are not at risk of dietary deficiency (such as calcium) by cutting out dairy foods over a longer period.

USEFUL ADDRESSES

Please send a stamped, self-addressed envelope if writing to any organization listed below for advice or information.

BRITISH DIGESTIVE FOUNDATION
3 St Andrew's Place
London NW1 4LB
Tel: 0171 487 5332

COELIAC SOCIETY
PO Box 220
High Wycombe
Bucks HP11 2HY
Tel: 01494 437278

IBS BULLETIN
Latest updates on diagnosis and treatment of IBS produced for sufferers by a team of medical researchers. For details of subscription send a sae to IBS Subscription Dept, Central Middlesex Hospital NHS Trust, PO Box 18, East Sussex TN6 1ZY.

The Central Middlesex Hospital NHS Trust IBS Research Team also runs a telephone Helpline: 0336 411286. At the time of writing, calls are 39p a minute cheap rate, 49p a minute at all other times.

IBS NETWORK
St John's House
Hither Green Hospital
London SE13 6RU
Tel: 0181 698 4611 ext. 8194

WOMEN'S NUTRITIONAL ADVISORY SERVICE
PO Box 268
Lewes
East Sussex BN7 2QN
Tel: 01273 487366
Advice and nutritional information for treating IBS

COMPLEMENTARY THERAPIES

BRITISH ACUPUNCTURE ASSOCIATION AND REGISTER
34 Alderney Street
London SW1V 4EU
Tel: 0171 834 1012
Information leaflets, booklets, register of qualified practitioners

BRITISH HERBAL MEDICINE ASSOCIATION
Sun House
Church Street
Stroud GL5 1JL
Tel: 01453 751389
Information leaflets, booklets, compendium, telephone advice

BRITISH HOMOEOPATHIC ASSOCIATION
27A Devonshire Street
London W1N 1RJ
Tel: 0171 935 2163
Leaflets, referral to medically qualified homoeopathic doctors

BRITISH SOCIETY OF MEDICAL AND DENTAL HYPNOTHERAPISTS
17 Keppel View Road
Kimberworth
Rotherham
South Yorks S61 2AR
Tel: 01709 554558

COLONIC IRRIGATIONS ASSOCIATION
50A Morrish Road
London SW2 4EG
Tel: 0181 671 7136

COUNCIL FOR COMPLEMENTARY AND ALTERNATIVE MEDICINE
Suite 1
19A Cavendish Square
London W1M 9AD
Tel: 0171 724 9103
Details on a variety of techniques and practices; leaflets, booklets, newsletter

GENERAL COUNCIL AND REGISTER OF NATUROPATHS
Frazer House
6 Netherall Gardens
London NW3 5RR
Tel: 0171 435 8728

INTERNATIONAL STRESS MANAGEMENT ASSOCIATION
The Priory Hospital
Priory Lane
London SW15 5JJ
Tel: 0181 876 8261
Information on stress management and control; leaflets, booklets, counselling

FURTHER READING

STRESS

Leon Chaitow. *Stress*, Thorsons, 1995
Robert Holden. *Stress Busters*, Thorsons, 1992
Stephen Terrass. *Stress*, Thorsons, 1994

ALTERNATIVE MEDICINE

Nicola M. Hall. *Principles of Reflexology*, Thorsons, 1996
David Hoffman. *The Complete Illustrated Holistic Herbal*,
   Element Books, 1996
Hellmut W. A. Karle. *Hypnotherapy*, Thorsons, 1988
Dr Andrew Lockie and Dr Nicola Geddes. *The Complete Guide to
   Homeopathy*, Dorling Kindersley, 1995
Dr Paul Marcus. *Acupuncture*, Thorsons, 1991
Penelope Ody. *The Herb Society's Complete Medicinal Herbal*,
   Dorling Kindersley, 1993
The Reader's Digest Family Guide to Alternative Medicine, 1991
Norman Shealy (ed.). *The Complete Family Guide to Alternative
   Medicine*, Element Books, 1996
Ronald Shone. *Creative Visualisation*, Thorsons, 1993
Dr Melvyn Werbach. *Healing through Nutrition*, Thorsons, 1995
Christine Wildwood. *The Aromatherapy and Massage Book*,
   Thorsons, 1994
Valerie Ann Worwood. *The Fragrant Pharmacy*,
   Bantam Books, 1991

INDEX

NuTron test 91

pain 29–30
peristalsis 4, 8, 16
piles *see* haemorrhoids
primary foregut motility
    disorder 11, 29
proctalgia fugax *see* rectal
    angina
proctoscopy 108
pulse testing 90

recipe:
    Apricot nut seed muesli 78
rectal:
    angina 41
    examination 105–106
    pain *see* rectal angina
    prolapse 35–6
reflexology 145
relaxants *see* anti-spasmodics
relaxation:
    deep 68–9
    general 68
Rome criteria 1–3
roughage *see* fibre

segmental contractions 16–17
silicic acid 145–6
skin:
    contact tests 90
    prick test 90
sleep and stress 71–4
sleep and herbs 73–4
small intestines 11–13
smoking 50–51
spastic:
    colitis *see* IBS – what it is
    colon *see* IBS – what it is

colon syndrome 28
constipation *see* IBS – what
    it is
stomach 10–11
stool:
    culture 107
    form and consistency 19–20
straining 20
stress: 53
    coping with 63–5
    diary 62–3
    and IBS 55
    and illness 57–8
    and large bowel 55
    and oesophagus 54
    and personality type 58–9
    and small intestine 54
    sources of 59–62
    and stomach 54
    what it is 55–7
stretching exercises
    (stress relief) 66–8
sublingual testing 89–90
surgery 126
sygmoidoscopy 108–9

transit studies 111

ultrasound 108
urgency 39

visualisation 146
vitamins and food intolerance
    93–5

wheat 87
wind 31–4

X-ray 108

Of further interest...

DIETS TO HELP COLITIS AND IBS

Natural relief with a carefully-balanced regime

JOAN LAY

Colitis, or inflammation of the colon, is a common ailment and sufferers experience frequent bouts of diarrhoea or constipation and stomach pains. The symptoms of irritable bowel syndrome are similar but often include abdominal bloating, wind, headaches and backaches. Feelings of stress only make matters worse and relief from both conditions lies in sufferers actively changing their lifestyles to restore health the natural way.

Includes:

- what causes colitis and irritable bowel syndrome
- a healing and cleansing programme that can help
- the importance of a carefully balanced diet

The author includes recipes and menu plans and advice on which foods will help and which to avoid.

IRRITABLE BOWEL SYNDROME & DIVERTICULOSIS

A self-help plan

SHIRLEY TRICKETT

Half the people who consult gastroenterologists with bowel problems are diagnosed as having Irritable Bowel Syndrome. Their symptoms vary – from chronic constipation to chronic diarrhoea, abdominal pains, colic, headaches and backache – and very often conventional treatment, such as high-fibre diets or drugs, makes matters worse. So, what exactly is IBS, and how can sufferers help themselves?

In straightforward style, Shirley Trickett explains the exact nature of the range of symptoms described as IBS, and what causes them. The effects of associated conditions such as Candidiasis, M.E., food allergies and addictions are described, and she provides practical suggestions for action in each case.

She then details a range of self-help therapies which can be of enormous benefit, including dietary changes, relaxation therapies, physical exercise and breathing techniques. Finally, the various approaches of several complementary therapies of proven benefit to bowel disorders – homoeopathy, therapeutic massage, colonic irrigation, reflexology, shiatsu and aromatherapy – are described by experts in each field.

BANISH ANXIETY

A common-sense plan for regaining control of your life

DR KENNETH HAMBLY

Do you feel anxious about work, your social life or even shopping?

It is perfectly normal and natural to react to difficult situations by becoming anxious. But do you feel you worry too much about things that you want to be able to cope with? Are you anxious all of the time? Do you experience excessive anxiety in difficult situations?

Dr Kenneth Hambly recognises that suffering from anxiety limits your life and prevents you from enjoying it to the full. He proposes a common-sense action plan for dealing with it and recovering from it.

By following Dr Hambly's advice, sufferers can regain a happier, healthier life and need never feel trapped by anxiety again.

HEALING THROUGH NUTRITION

**A natural approach to treating 50 common illnesses
with diet and nutrients**

DR MELVYN R. WERBACH

This indispensable reference book provides the nutritional roots
of and treatments for 50 common illnesses, from allergies and
the common cold to cancer.

The world's authority on the relationship between nutrition
and illness, Dr Melvyn Werbach makes it easy to learn what
you can do to influence the course of your health via the nutrients that you feed your body.

A chapter is devoted to each of the 50 ailments and this highly accessible A-Z of nutritional health includes:

- an analysis of dietary factors affecting health and well-being
- a suggested healing diet for 50 common illnesses
- nutritional healing plans, with recommended dosages for
  vitamins, minerals and other essential nutrients
- an explanation of vitamin supplements and how they can
  improve your health

There are also guidelines on how to plan the right healing diet
for yourself and how to diagnose food sensitivities. With this
groundbreaking guide you will be able to make informed decisions about the essential role of nutrients in your health and
well-being.

STRESS

Proven stress-coping strategies for better health

LEON CHAITOW

Do you suffer from migraine, chronic back pain, frequent colds, fatigue, panic attacks or high blood pressure? If so, you could be suffering from stress which can damage your health.

Stress has a disastrous effect on our immune systems, and can be the major cause of both mild and serious health problems. Psychoneuroimmunology, or PNI, is the science which holds the key to many common health problems. It points to new ways in which damaging emotions can be controlled, so protecting our bodies' natural defences and warding off illness.

Leading health writer, Leon Chaitow, uses the latest research into the mind/body connection to help you create your own stress protection plan. Advice on diet, exercise, meditation, relaxation, guided imagery and visualization, with useful checklists, will help you develop your own system to cope with the inevitable pressures of everyday life.

THE BOOK OF PAIN RELIEF

LEON CHAITOW

Pain is the body's warning signal, a vital protective mechanism which alerts us that something is wrong. Chronic pain, however, serves no useful purpose and can trigger other physical and emotional problems, while long-term use of medication can make the underlying problem worse. Health expert Leon Chaitow explains how to break the never-ending cycle of pain, medication and misery, so that pain is eased or even removed altogether.

This definitive guide to how pain may affect any part of the body allows you to discover what's right for you; many beneficial treatments can be carried out at home, and the practical solutions include:

- self-help methods for immediate relief
- how to release the body's own natural pain-killers
- how dietary changes can help
- acupuncture, electrotherapy and massage
- herbal remedies, homoeopathy and aromatherapy
- the benefits of water treatment
- healing and therapeutic touch
- the role of relaxation and stress reduction

This is an empowering book that will help us regain control of our bodies and our lives.

DIETS TO HELP COLITIS AND IBS	0 7225 3199 0	£2.99	☐
IRRITABLE BOWEL SYNDROME & DIVERTICULOSIS	0 7225 2401 3	£5.99	☐
BANISH ANXIETY	0 7225 3112 5	£5.99	☐
HEALING THROUGH NUTRITION	0 7225 2941 4	£16.99	☐
STRESS	0 7225 3192 3	£5.99	☐
BOOK OF PAIN RELIEF	0 7225 2820 5	£7.99	☐

All these books are available from your local bookseller or can be ordered direct from the publishers.

To order direct just tick the titles you want and fill in the form below:

Name: _____

Address: _____

_____ Postcode: _____

Send to Thorsons Mail Order, Dept 3, HarperCollinsPublishers, Westerhill Road, Bishopbriggs, Glasgow G64 2QT.

Please enclose a cheque or postal order or your authority to debit your Visa/Access account —

Credit card no: _____

Expiry date: _____

Signature: _____

— up to the value of the cover price plus:

UK & BFPO: Add £1.00 for the first book and 25p for each additional book ordered.

Overseas orders including Eire: Please add £2.95 service charge. Books will be sent by surface mail but quotes for airmail dispatches will be given on request.

24-HOUR TELEPHONE ORDERING SERVICE FOR ACCESS/VISA CARDHOLDERS — TEL: 0141 772 2281.